Praise for *Healthy Eating, Hea...*

"J. Morris Hicks has done us all a tremendous se... a simple, clear, and profoundly helpful guide t... erful benefits of plant-strong nutrition. If you want to be healthy, read this amazing book. In a world hungry for hope, this book arrives at precisely the right time." —JOHN ROBBINS, bestselling author
The Food Revolution and *Diet For A New America*

"*Healthy Eating, Healthy World* is more than an eye-opening, fact-filled book about the causes of poor health. It is a map leading directly to the cure. In the process, it points the way toward solving the seemingly unrelated problems of environmental destruction and world hunger. It is sensible, direct, and right." —NEAL D. BARNARD, MD,
President, Physicians Committee for Responsible Medicine

"What's good for you is also good for our planet. Although heart disease and diabetes kill more people each year worldwide than all other diseases combined, these are completely preventable and even reversible for at least 95% of people today by changing our diet and lifestyle. This book shows you how." —DEAN ORNISH, MD,
Founder, Preventive Medicine Research Institute;
Clinical Professor of Medicine, University of California, San Francisco;
and author of *The Spectrum* and *Dr. Dean Ornish's Program for Reversing Heart Disease*

"*Healthy Eating, Healthy World* is by far one of my favorite books. It is incredibly informative, well researched, and a must read for anyone who eats! It takes you on a journey towards adopting a plant-based diet in a way that isn't overwhelming and provides much needed tips about eating this way for good." —KIM BARNOUIN, co-author
of the #1 *New York Times* bestseller *Skinny Bitch*

"Poor nutrition is our leading cause of disease. Yet the biggest impediment to improving our health is that most people mistakenly believe they are eating a good diet. With the costs of disease out of control and threatening the economic health of our country, *Healthy Eating, Healthy World* is a timely contribution, explaining in clear, easy-to-read language why our standard diet is making us sick, and how you can make simple choices that will improve your health, longevity and quality of life. This is a must-read book. Highly recommended!" —RAYMOND FRANCIS, MS (from MIT),
scientist and bestselling author of *Never Be Sick Again*

"The same standard diet-style, rich in processed foods and animal products, and low in produce, that places people at high risk of heart attacks and cancers, is also rapidly destroying our environment. *Healthy Eating, Healthy World* reports on critical information you must learn to help ourselves and our planet." —JOEL FUHRMAN, MD, family physician and author of the bestselling *Eat to Live*

"J. Morris Hicks's world-changing book, *Healthy Eating, Healthy World*, is compelling in transforming our health—promoting dietary choices to be over 80% from whole plant foods. Not only will we restore our own fitness, vigor and happiness as we become healthier; we will be celebrating a world-wide paradigm shift by living in harmony with nature on our precious planet." —ALEXANDRA STODDARD, author of bestselling *Living a Beautiful Life* and twenty-six other books

"Reading and implementing *Healthy Eating, Healthy World* is the best prescription you will ever fill."
—HOWARD F. LYMAN, LLD, author of *Mad Cowboy*

"In *Healthy Eating, Healthy World*, the title tells it all, as author Jim Hicks masterfully resolves global challenges in a sensible, well-written, highly referenced must-read."
—CALDWELL B. ESSELSTYN, JR., MD,
Director of Cardiovascular Disease Prevention and Reversal
at the Wellness Institute of The Cleveland Clinic,
and author of *Prevent & Reverse Heart Disease*

"We all know we should eat more fruits and vegetables—with this book, we now know why. The authors make a well-documented case for why it is important for your personal health and why it is critical for the health of the planet. A compelling book; it is both informative and a pleasure to read!" —PAUL ALLAIRE,
Fortune 100 CEO (Xerox, 1990-1999)

HEALTHY EATING
HEALTHY WORLD

UNLEASHING THE POWER OF PLANT-BASED NUTRITION

J. MORRIS HICKS

WITH J. STANFIELD HICKS

FOREWORD BY

T. COLIN CAMPBELL, PHD, AND NELSON CAMPBELL

BENBELLA BOOKS, INC. | DALLAS, TEXAS

BenBella Books, Inc.
10300 N. Central Expressway
Suite #400
Dallas, TX 75231
www.benbellabooks.com
Send feedback to feedback@benbellabooks.com

Printed in the United States of America
10 9 8 7 6 5 4 3 2 1

Library of Congress Cataloging-in-Publication Data is available for this title.
ISBN : 978-1-936661-04-6

Editing by Erin Kelley
Copyediting by Rebecca Logan
Proofreading by Michael Fedison and Nora Nussbaum
Cover design by Kit Sweeney
Text design and composition by Neuwirth & Associates
Printed by Bang Printing

Distributed by Perseus Distribution
perseusdistribution.com

To place orders through Perseus Distribution:
Tel: 800-343-4499
Fax: 800-351-5073
E-mail: orderentry@perseusbooks.com

Significant discounts for bulk sales are available. Please contact Glenn Yeffeth at glenn@benbellabooks.com or (214) 750-3628.

To the memory of my father,
Morris Adron Hicks,
whose constant positive reinforcement,
during the beginning of my quest to learn the truth about
nutrition, led me to discover and explore a much bigger
picture than I ever imagined.

And to the memory of my mother,
Agnes Stanfield Hicks,
whose unconditional love, support, and confidence
during my early years planted in me a compelling desire to do
something meaningful with my life and whose
suggestion that I take a typing class in the eleventh grade,
instead of wasting my time in study hall,
made the physical task of writing this book so much easier.

ACKNOWLEDGMENTS

The origins of this book go back to the Peachtree Presbyterian Church of Atlanta and the Georgia Tech Alumni Association—both of whom played a key role in my receiving an invitation to speak on the Tech campus in 2002. As a result of the reaction to that speech, I became very curious about nutrition—specifically, the optimal diet for humans.

That curiosity led to five years of intensive study. While I learned from hundreds of people, I was influenced most by T. Colin Campbell, PhD; Caldwell Esselstyn, Jr., MD; and Joel Fuhrman, MD. I met all three in 2005 at the Zen Palate restaurant in New York City (and I thank Caryn Hartglass and the people at EarthSave for organizing events such as the one that brought about our meeting). Other MDs who contributed mightily to my body of knowledge were John McDougall, Neal Barnard, and Dean Ornish. I also acknowledge that the authors of *Fit for Life*, Harvey and Marilyn Diamond, initially planted the seeds of my interest in nutrition way back in 1989.

Six months into my quest for learning in 2003, I read two powerful books—one by John Robbins (*Diet for a New America*) and the other by Howard Lyman (*Mad Cowboy*). Until then, my interest was primarily on the relationship between diet and health, but their books raised other food-related issues—crucial issues such as the environment, energy, world hunger, and the suffering of animals. It was a *blinding flash of the obvious* as the natural diet for our species became crystal clear to me for the first time.

Then there's my friend Bo Rinaldi, who introduced me to my agent, Marilyn Allen, who secured the contracts with my publisher and with my editor. It was those partnerships with Glenn Yeffeth and his team at BenBella Books and my editor, John Paine, that made this book a reality. Also, quite a few of my business friends have made important contributions along the way: Susan Benigas, Gina Copeland, Nelson Campbell, Bob Pravder, and Kevin Leville.

My personal friends and family have helped in countless ways. For all their unconditional love, encouragement, and support, I thank my siblings, Sherrill, Carol, Paul, and Virginia. And for a number of special reasons, I thank Nigel Richardson, Shawn Lankton, Clark Seydel, Bob Wyatt, Laura Moran, Mary Elliott, Peter Megargee Brown, and Alexandra Stoddard.

I especially thank Ruth Seydel for bringing me to that church mentioned previously and for her suggestion long ago that I become a professional speaker. I greatly appreciate Tom Dickey, my good friend of over forty-five years, for his brutal honesty regarding the all-important tone and voice of this book. I also thank my favorite bartender, Karen Cochran, and restaurant owners, Stephanie and Walter Houlihan, who have joyfully facilitated my learning how to order a healthy meal in any fine restaurant—such as their Water Street Café in Stonington, Connecticut.

Finally, I want to thank my two children. I owe gratitude to my daughter, Diana Shewchuk, for the steady and positive inspiration she has always provided. And I thank my son and cowriter, Jason, and his wife, Lisa, who are living proof of the magic of the wonderful diet style described in these pages. Their enthusiastic participation in this project has been essential.

J. Morris Hicks

CONTENTS

FOREWORD

By T. Colin Campbell, PhD, and Nelson Campbell

Most of us live apart from Nature, within artificially constructed environments that bear little resemblance to the mountains, meadows, forests and streams experienced by our ancestors. And living apart from Nature, we too often forget that we are part of an interconnected whole.

No matter how hard we try, however, we cannot escape this fact forever. We can construct our material world and engage in individualistic pursuits, but eventually must face the fact that we do not live on islands. We are connected to one another and to the larger natural world of which we are still a part.

There may be no better illustration of this truth than the way we eat. The decision of what to put at the end of our fork is a private decision and one that seems to have no relevance beyond the edges of our dinner plate. But the truth is this: the effects of what we eat ripple round and round the world . . . and this is the story of *Healthy Eating, Healthy World* by J. Morris Hicks.

When Jim approached us about writing the foreword for this book, we did not hesitate to answer his call. Jim is a good friend, but more than a friend—he is an intelligent man whose life experiences have prepared him well for this moment. Trained as a strategy and process improvement consultant, he has spent much of his professional career helping organizations understand and improve the quality of their operations, services and products. He is trained to see the world from a "big picture" systems perspective, so it was not hard for him to grasp the interconnections between what we eat and our broader world and how we might make changes within this system to improve the quality of our lives.

Too often in a field of study, we rely solely on those people who have established themselves as the inside "experts." Yet, sometimes the most interesting perspectives are those that come from outside the field. And this is the case here—Jim's perspective has enabled him to tell a story in *Healthy Eating, Healthy World* that is informative, engaging, and compelling.

While told from a "systems" perspective, this story also is one of *personal empowerment*. As it turns out, what is best for the system is also best for our individual health. When we consume a whole food plant-based diet, with minimal additions of fat, salt, sugar and other refined ingredients, we optimize a larger system encompassing economics, politics, and the environment, while also optimizing the internal system that gives us life.

This is a powerful idea with a bright future. The idea that we can control our health largely by what we eat offers a bright light within a seemingly dimly lit world. We often feel out of control, not always because we are out of control, but because the world we live within feels increasingly out of control. So the idea that we can take charge of what is most precious to us, our personal well-being, is a powerful idea indeed.

And many of us are more open to transformative social change than ever before. Population growth, rapid technological development, environmental destruction, and increasing economic and political control in the hands of people who have forgotten the old-fashioned idea of civic virtue, all have propelled us to a point in human history where the acceptable margin for error has become a thin line. There is an urgency that exists today that did not exist in years past, and it is this sense of urgency that will open people to the story of this book.

J. Morris Hicks and his son have put together an interesting tale that will enlighten you while also giving you great hope. The message of plant-based nutrition already has transformed many lives, including the life of this management consultant and former senior corporate executive. Not only has he put himself and his family on a path to optimal health, he has also become so passionate about the idea that he has launched a new career to share this good news with others. That new career features a blend of speaking, blogging, consulting and writing—all beginning with this powerful book that you hold in your hands.

—T. Colin Campbell, PhD, and Nelson Campbell

Dr. T. Colin Campbell, author of The China Study, *is the foremost science expert in the field of plant-based nutrition and is working with his son, Nelson, who is coordinating an effort to develop and implement a strategy for promoting the message of plant-based nutrition into the mainstream.*

INTRODUCTION

"It turns out that if we eat the way that promotes the best health for ourselves, we also promote the best health for the planet."

—T. Colin Campbell, PhD, author of *The China Study*

Millions of creatures have evolved throughout the ages on our planet, and until recently, they have all lived in harmony with nature. During the past few hundred years—a mere blink of the eye in history—one species has unknowingly thrown the natural scheme out of balance. That species is us—the human race. Although we mean no harm for ourselves, for the planet, or for the other creatures, we have drifted far away from the natural diet for our species. We have started eating the wrong food—in great quantities. This change in diet has set in motion a series of chain reactions that has negatively affected the planet in many ways.

Our craving for the rich Western diet has intensified to the point that we have almost totally abandoned the type of fuel that nature intended for us to burn. Whereas animals in the wild with DNA closest to ours consume almost 100 percent raw plants, the humans of the Western world today are consuming virtually none. We now consume generous portions of meat, dairy, eggs and/or highly processed foods three meals a day and are deriving far less than 10 percent of our calories from whole plant foods. In addition, many of the plants that we do eat are french fries, which gain over 40 percent of their calories from the fat in the oil in which they are prepared.[1] This love affair with a very unhealthy diet has begun taking its toll in myriad ways both within our bodies and without, affecting the world.

In the United States and other Western countries, obesity and diabetes are running rampant, while heart disease and cancer maintain their position as our top killers—and the top drivers of our health-care costs. These out-of-control costs are choking our economy to death, prompting elected officials in the United States to frequently discuss health-care cost as the single biggest problem facing our nation. In 1960, the cost of health care in the Unites States was 5.2 percent of the gross domestic product (GDP). In less than fifty years, it tripled to 16 percent, and U.S. officials now project that it will double again to 31 percent within the next twenty-five years.[2] This cost is simply unsustainable, and we all know it, but we haven't yet figured out what can be done to address the problem.

It turns out that much of this health-care problem is food-driven. We are eating way too much of the wrong food. What is the optimal diet for humans? It's one based on what your mother may have told you long ago: "You should eat more fruits and vegetables." We rarely hear health officials, doctors, dietitians, or nutritionists advising us to eat more meat, dairy, or processed foods. They're all saying we should eat more vegetables, but with each passing year, we seem to be eating fewer. Why is that? The first part of the book explores this question, outlines the many health benefits of an optimal diet and addresses various arguments against the adoption of such a diet.

But health is just one of the issues. What you eat affects far more than just your body. You may already know about some of the environmental impacts of our rich Western diet, but you may not have heard much about other related problems, such as the rising cost and decreasing availability of energy (especially fossil fuels), the increasingly difficult challenge of feeding the growing population of the world, and the horrific suffering of 60 billion animals per year in the factory farms where they are raised. The second part of the book is devoted to an exploration of these four categories of critical global issues.

At some point during your reading, you may very well ask yourself, "Why haven't I heard all this before?" That is a very good question, inviting us to look at the vast system that controls the flow of this kind of information in our society. The third part of the book explores this question in detail, helping you to digest all that you have read and decide how you will act on that information. Whatever you choose for you and your family, this book can help you execute your plan, providing you with information, helpful tips, and guidelines that you may need to reach your goals.

In a nutshell, this book is about the single most powerful move that we humans can make to promote health, reduce obesity, lower the cost of health care, nurture our fragile environment, conserve our energy resources, feed the world's steadily growing population, and greatly reduce the suffering of animals in factory farms all over the world. This move is an aggressive push to consume more whole, plant-based foods—not necessarily becoming a vegetarian or a vegan. These "v" words only convey information about what a person does *not* eat; they do little to convey what the person *does* eat, and that is what is most important. A great many vegetarians eat an unhealthy diet and, as a result, fail to enjoy the host of benefits that result from eating a truly health-promoting diet. After all, one could consume nothing but Diet Coke and potato chips and call himself a vegan.

What about weight loss? While this is not specifically a weight-loss book, adopting a diet of whole plant foods will enable your body to seek its ideal weight effortlessly and permanently. Many health professionals and researchers cite the statistic that diets fail 95 percent of the time.[3] Compare that to a near 100 percent success rate for those who make a commitment to a health-promoting diet for the right reasons—to achieve vibrant health. When vibrant health is your primary objective, effortless weight loss is simply a convenient by-product or fringe benefit.

The primary objective of this book is to outline in simple, everyday terms the extent of the problems we face, how we got ourselves into trouble, and what each of us can do to make things better. Fortunately, despite the incredible complexity of our current dilemma, the solution is refreshingly simple. All we have to do is educate ourselves, start making better choices about what we eat, and then share all that we have learned with everyone we care about. I am convinced that there has never been anything more important in the history of the world.

"Chase perfection. Settle for excellence along the way."

—Vince Lombardi, *What It Takes to Be #1*

PART I

You Are What You Eat

1

WHAT SHOULD WE BE EATING?

> "You put a baby in a crib with an apple and a rabbit. If it eats the rabbit and plays with the apple, I'll buy you a new car."
>
> —Harvey Diamond, author of *Fit for Life*

A friend of mine, Eric Williams, is trying to eat healthy. He has heard that red meat has more fat and cholesterol, so he has cut down on it in favor of chicken and fish. He has vegetables along with the main course, because he read that he needed to eat a balanced diet. He doesn't eat chips much anymore, and the only sweets he allows himself are a few Chips Ahoys after a meal. Being healthy is good, but giving up chocolate is taking things a little too far. He exercises some, giving the dog a walk every morning before work, and he plays golf when he's not away traveling on the weekend. In other words, Eric is not some balloon figure chowing down burgers by the backyard barbeque. He wants to live a long time.

Yet Eric is thirty pounds overweight. He has been taking medication for high blood pressure for over twenty years. He often feels tired after lunch, and he wishes he had a couch in his office so he could lie down for a five-minute power nap. He used to play tennis with a group of friends, but the last time he played, his heart clutched up and he started seeing spots in front of his eyes. These days he lives with a constant, nagging worry. He knows that many men have heart attacks around age fifty. He is afraid that he'll have a massive stroke, paralyzing one side of his body, making him a vegetable for the rest of his life. He is trying, really trying, so why isn't he seeing any results?

Eric's situation is far from uncommon. Most people in the developed world eat a typical Western diet that features animal products three meals a day, 365 days a year. While humans have always craved calorie-dense foods like meat, oil, and cheese, they were simply not available or affordable in great quantities until about sixty or seventy years ago. That is when these types of foods began to be mass-produced and distributed so efficiently that nowadays billions of people can easily afford to eat them. As these foods became common, everyday people began to experience the diseases that had previously attacked only the affluent class.

In the past, only royalty and the very rich could afford these rich foods. They suffered from obesity, heart disease, diabetes, cancer, osteoporosis, and other diseases that came to be known as the "diseases of affluence." Conversely, in less advanced populations where most people primarily ate whole, plant-based foods, these diseases were almost nonexistent. But not anymore. With the exportation of our rich Western diet to Japan, China, India, and other countries, their people have begun to experience the same levels of those diseases as the United States and Europe.

We have been eating this way for so long now that many of us think we eat a pretty healthy diet and that we can improve our health if we simply "watch what we eat." Most people who work in the vast industries that create our food supply actually believe they are providing nourishment; they are just doing what they have been taught. The truth is that the typical Western diet contains very little nutrition. In August 2010, the *New York Times* cited a report from the Centers for Disease Control and Prevention (CDC) saying that Americans were continuing to get fatter and fatter, with obesity rates reaching 30 percent or more in nine states in 2009, as opposed to only three states in 2007. Obesity rates have doubled in adults and tripled in children in recent decades, said Dr. Thomas Frieden, director of the CDC.[4] The following is a summary of information on the global obesity epidemic from a 2008 World Health Organization fact sheet.

- Worldwide obesity has more than doubled since 1980.
- There are more than 1.5 billion overweight adults in the world; at least 500 million of them are obese.
- Both conditions pose a major risk for chronic disease, including type 2 diabetes, cardiovascular disease, stroke, and certain forms of cancer.
- Key causes are increased consumption of energy-dense foods high in saturated fats and sugars and reduced physical activity.
- Obesity rates have risen threefold or more since 1980 in some areas of North America, Europe, the Middle East, and China.
- Current obesity levels range from below 5 percent in China, Japan, and certain African nations to over 75 percent in urban Samoa.
- Even in countries with a relatively low prevalence, like China, rates are almost 20 percent in some cities.[5]

Many scientists have now drawn a link between obesity and heart disease, the number-one killer in the United States and a pressing problem all over the Western world. According to the CDC, we're not winning the war against heart disease either. "In 2006 . . . heart disease caused 26% of deaths—more than one in every four—in the United States. In 2010, heart disease will cost the United States $316.4 billion. This total includes the cost of health-care services, medications, and lost productivity."[6]

The link between obesity and diabetes has also become common knowledge, and this medical problem has become positively frightening.

The *New York Times* reported in October 2009, "Among Americans 30 and older, 13.7 percent of men and 11.9 percent of women have diabetes. Almost one-third of them have never received a diagnosis of the disease."[7] Type 2 diabetes (formerly called adult-onset diabetes) has reached epidemic proportions in the United States. According to the *Times* in January 2006, "One in three children born in the United States five years ago are expected to become diabetic in their lifetimes, according to a projection by the Centers for Disease Control and Prevention."[8] Even more worrying, the problem is now directly affecting our youth. The article continues, "So-called Type 2 diabetes, the predominant form . . . , is creeping into children, something almost unheard of two decades ago. The American Diabetes Association says the disease could actually lower the average life expectancy of Americans for the first time in more than a century."[9]

But even as the frequency and related costs of our chronic diseases continue to rise, there is hope on the horizon. In the past thirty or forty years, an innovative group of doctors and scientists have been creating revolutionary treatments for arresting and even reversing these terrible modern plagues. Surprisingly, their paradigm has not been based on new drugs or new breakthroughs in surgical techniques. They have focused on diet. Hippocrates, known as the father of medicine, is reported to have said several thousand years ago: "Your food will be your medicine, and your medicine will be your food." He was referring to the human body's ability to promote health as long as we feed it the right stuff. It's not that hard if we understand how our bodies really function.

The Way We Were

In those wonderful illustrated books from our childhood, one common picture is of a group of hairy cave people gathered around a large beast that they have slain with mere stone arrows and clubs. While it is true that early humans would eat anything that came their way, they didn't live off ancient steak as their primary source of food. As is well known, humankind hunted and gathered nuts and berries and, primarily, plants. Nature's bounty provided them with all they needed to develop into a more intelligent species.

In short, we are natural herbivores, not carnivores. So how did we grow big and strong without a regular diet of animal protein? One clue comes from animals most like humans, such as gorillas and chimpanzees. They primarily eat raw plants, and that doesn't seem to stunt their growth. A male silverback can weigh over 400 pounds. The fact that their DNA is among the closest to that of humans should give us a pretty good idea what we should be eating. Many of the other strongest animals in the world (elephants, giraffes, horses, etc.) also eat nothing but raw plants. They know something that modern man seems to have forgotten. Plants have plenty of protein.

We don't need to search through the mists of time, though, for people who eat mainly a plant-based diet. Even today we can find less-advanced cultures that cannot afford to eat meat. Their diet consists primarily of whole, unrefined plant foods and very little, if any, animal products. Heart disease, cancer, diabetes, and other diseases of affluence are almost nonexistent in these whole-plant-eating cultures. In his book *Healthy at 100*, John Robbins documented the current diet of three separate long-lived cultures—the peoples of Abkhasia in Russia, Vilcabamba in Ecuador, and Hunza in Pakistan. Their consumption of plant-based foods is 99 percent for two of the cultures and 90 percent for the other. All three cultures consume zero processed foods, derive 20 percent or less of their calories from fat, and have zero incidence of obesity.[10] In contrast, the average American gets far less than 10 percent of his or her calories from whole plants and close to 40 percent from fat.[11]

In November 2008, *National Geographic* featured an article on a fourth primitive culture that shares much in common with the other three—the Tarahumara tribe, who live in and above the canyons of northern Mexico's Sierra Madre Occidental, where they retreated in the sixteenth century to avoid invading Spaniards. These primitive people, who are famous for their athletic prowess in long-distance running, live on a diet consisting almost exclusively of corn, beans, and squash. A recent *Men's Health* article dubbed them "The Men Who Live Forever" and described them as "a tribe of Indians that carries an ancient secret: a diet and fitness regimen that has allowed them to outrun death and disease . . . When it comes to the top 10 health risks facing American men, the Tarahumara are practically immortal: Their incidence rate is at or near zero in just about every category, including diabetes, vascular disease, and colorectal cancer."[12]

If you look at American and European records, you'll also see that the major diseases of today hardly existed for most of our history. Although human farming techniques evolved over the millennia, we continued to eat much as our earliest forebears did right up until the nineteenth century. At that time, people were far more worried about influenza and tuberculosis. The idea of counting calories would have been laughable. But our diet began to change. In the nineteenth century, revolutionary advances such as Cyrus McCormick's mechanical reaper permitted farmers to greatly expand crop production. The movement toward today's diet accelerated with the completion of the transcontinental railroads. For the first time, beef, pork, and wheat could be transported to mushrooming city populations. Surrounding the cities, market gardening and dairy farms proliferated. Housewives were soon encouraged to buy labor-saving processed foods such as canned goods. That trend gained momentum after World War II, when frozen foods and other new kinds of processed, precooked, and packaged foods became popular. Chemists developed more than 400 additives to help food survive these new processes—and make it taste good. By the mid-1970s, the boom in takeout foods began, as did eating out, particularly at fast-food and other chain restaurants.[13]

Today all these developments are regarded as facts of life. According to the USDA Economic Research Service, the per capita consumption of meat continues to increase—rising sharply from 144 pounds in 1950 to 222 pounds in 2007.[14] Within the same period, the consumption of cheese grew at a much faster rate. It skyrocketed 193 percent from 1976 to 2001—a period of rapid growth of delivery pizza and fast-food restaurants.[15]

Paralleling this growth in meat and cheese consumption in the United States has been the spread of the American diet, especially the explosion of fast-food restaurants worldwide. In 2005, Eric Schlosser in *Fast Food Nation* observed: "A decade ago, McDonald's had about three thousand restaurants outside the United States; today it has about seventeen thousand restaurants in more than 120 foreign countries."[16] The first decade of the new millennium, which witnessed a massive growth in globalization, was good for the fast-food industry as well; there are now more than 31,000 McDonald's restaurants worldwide, serving some 58 million customers daily.

Why Do We Like Foods That Are Not Good for Us?

If the whole, plant-based foods that we used to eat are the most nutritious, why do we crave many foods that we know are not good for us? Did Mother Nature play a trick on us? Why did she let that happen? Doug Lisle and Alan Goldhamer do a great job of explaining this mystery in *The Pleasure Trap: Mastering the Hidden Force That Undermines Health and Happiness*. They explain that all species have two essential purposes: to survive and reproduce. To aid us in achieving these goals, nature provided all species with what Lisle and Goldhamer call a "motivational triad"—a tendency to seek pleasure, avoid pain, and conserve energy.[17] Like the gorillas, our early ancestors ate mostly plants, but, having been blessed with a cognitive niche (the ability to reason), man taught himself how to kill, cook, and eat other animals and fish. Lisle and Goldhamer sum it up: "For hundreds of thousands of years, our human ancestors struggled to survive. While our ancient ancestors faced many adaptive challenges—injury, disease, and periodic tribal warfare—their greatest challenge was getting enough to eat."[18] In the wild, our ancestors instinctively ate things that looked and tasted good to them, or whatever food that they could gather or kill. They naturally preferred calorically dense nuts, avocados, and meat as they sought pleasure, avoided pain, and conserved energy. So why didn't they eat too much of the high-fat foods? These foods simply weren't available in great quantities.

Fast-forward to the twentieth century. Animal foods that were eaten only on rare, festive occasions gradually became more available—so much so that by the end of that century, the typical Western diet provided several forms of animal foods at almost every meal. So when your child says that he prefers pizza to broccoli, he is just following his natural motivational triad. He doesn't yet know that cheese-laden pizza is not good for his health; he just knows that he likes it. This is what the "pleasure trap" is all about. We're following our natural instinct to seek pleasure, but we're exercising this instinct in an unnatural world—a world full of unhealthy choices everywhere we go.

So, according to Lisle and Goldhamer, it is no wonder that people have eaten too much of the wrong foods. But once they realize they've fallen into the pleasure trap, they can exercise that special feature that is exclusive to the human race—their *cognitive niche*—and they must take responsibility for their own actions.

What Role Do Our Genes Play?

With the completion of the mapping of the human genome, a new question has entered the discussion about the causes of modern-day diseases. Is the problem all in our genes? Am I doomed, no matter what I do, if I have a family history of, for instance, pancreatic cancer?

The reason these new questions are being asked is because scientists are discovering more and more genes that are linked with the major diseases. Every week, it seems, a new announcement is made about a discovery of a genetic link. These findings have created a whole new level of fear in the general populace. For instance, the knowledge of a family history of breast cancer has led some women to have radical mastectomies (removal of the entire breast) even before a mammogram shows they have cancer. But this automatic association has some basic problems. First, not everyone who has a family member with cancer ends up dying from cancer. How does the predisposition skip one person and mark the next? The second problem lies in the scientific method. We still know very little about our genetic makeup. In some ways, the hunt for genetic markers of different diseases is the scientific equivalent of the magic bullet: if we can only isolate and then snip out that defective marker, the entire disease will vanish. This belief is far too simplistic.

The difficulty involved in linking markers to disease is illustrated in *The China Study*, the best-selling book based on 27 years of research on 170 different villages in China and Taiwan. Its author, T. Colin Campbell, makes this point about genetics: "Recently, for example, researchers studied genetic regulation of weight in a tiny worm species. The scientists went through 16,757 genes, turning each one off, and observed the effect on weight. They discovered 417 genes that affect weight. How these hundreds of genes interact over the long term with each other and their ever-changing environment to alter weight gain or loss is an incredibly complex mystery."[19]

We can look at the question of genetic makeup in another way. Do the genes of a certain race play a role in their susceptibility to diseases? Here the answer is much clearer. There are numerous examples of groups that eat both Western and non-Western diets, and they disprove the idea that some people have better genes than others. Dr. John McDougall, author of *The McDougall Program for a Healthy Heart*, discovered this early in his medical career. He treated five generations of Chinese, Japanese, and Filipinos working on plantations in Hawaii. "What I saw was that the older generation who had continued to follow their traditional eating patterns had none of the heart disease, high blood pressure, cancer, arthritis, and intestinal disorders that their children had. At first, this baffled me, until I began to ask family members what they were eating."[20] It turned out that the older generation still didn't eat meat or dairy products, while their Hawaiian-born children and grandchildren were eating the standard American diet—hamburgers, french fries, potato chips, and the like.

In another example, the data suggest that genes do not affect our health as much as environment. According to studies reported by the *Journal of the National Cancer Institute (JNCI)* in 2006, "Most breast cancer cases occur in industrialized countries in Europe and North America, whereas the disease is less common among developing countries in Africa and Asia."[21] As with other diseases of affluence, breast cancer rates are much higher in the countries where people eat the typical Western diet and much lower in the more primitive cultures in which people consume more whole plant foods. The *JNCI* report continues, "Over the past four decades, many studies have shown that breast cancer rates change when women move to a new country, providing evidence for the importance of lifestyle and environment in breast cancer risk."[22] Studies of this type are called migrant studies. "Migration provides a kind of natural experiment allowing the comparison of populations of similar genetic background living in different environments," said Max Parkin, an epidemiologist at the University of Oxford in the United Kingdom. One study noted in the *JNCI* report compared breast cancer incidence rates of Japanese women who migrated to Los Angeles, San Francisco, and Hawaii to the rates of Japanese women still living in Japan. The incidence rates on average for the American cities were more than twice as high as the rates for Japanese women living in Japan. A separate study showed that the third generation of Asian American women living in the United States has rates similar to or greater than white women in the United States.[23]

Even within the same country, examples of the link between Western-based diets and obesity can be found. The most glaring example is in China, which for decades was closed off to the outside world. Once it started modernizing, its people, particularly in cities, started eating Western food. The changes were sudden and startling. In 2004, BBC News reported that the incidence of obesity in China had increased by 97 percent between 1992 and 2002.[24] This increase correlates with rises in rates of cancer, heart disease, and diabetes, also concentrated in the cities.[25]

The same changes can be found all across the globe. The World Health Organization recently reported:

> Increased consumption of more energy-dense, nutrient-poor foods with high levels of sugar and saturated fats, combined with reduced physical activity, have led to obesity rates that have risen three-fold or more since 1980 in some areas of North America, the United Kingdom, Eastern Europe, the Middle East, the Pacific Islands, Australasia and China. The obesity epidemic is not restricted to industrialized societies; this increase is often faster in developing countries than in the developed world.[26]

Breakthroughs in Defense of Our Health

Luckily, help is on the horizon. As has happened so often in the course of history, when the pendulum swings too far to one extreme—in this case, the horrific toll of these modern diseases—nature finds a counterbalance. As these diseases became more common, doctors were confronted with patients afflicted with these problems and felt a responsibility to solve them. Over the past century, and particularly in the past thirty years, doctors and scientists have discovered new techniques that have produced highly positive results.

The idea that nutrition promotes good health is not new. Hippocrates referred to it as early as 400 BC, and medical people knew about the link long before the Western diet evolved into the three feasts a day that are driving the current obesity and health-care dilemmas. Physicians in the first half of the twentieth century cured patients in sanitariums with natural diets and with fasting. One of those physicians was Herbert Shelton, who was one of the earliest doctors to accept alternative medicine.

In the second half of the twentieth century, our Western diet began to get much worse. During the 1970s, about the time that our rich Western diet was becoming widespread in the United States and Europe, a few truth-seeking pioneers began searching for a better way to treat patients—focusing on the cause of the disease instead of the symptoms. This section profiles these doctors.

Caldwell Esselstyn, Jr., MD. An Olympic gold medalist, winner of a bronze star in Vietnam, and one of the top-billing surgeons in the history of the highly respected Cleveland Clinic, this man is the real deal—and will likely be recognized someday as a true American hero. In the early 1970s, while working as a general surgeon at the Cleveland Clinic, Esselstyn became disenchanted with the conventional treatment paradigm for cancer, heart disease, and diabetes. While spending most of his time conducting surgical procedures such as mastectomies two or three times daily, he became troubled that his medical team was not addressing the root causes of the patients' problems. Not wanting to become known as the man who had disfigured more women than anyone in the state of Ohio, he began conducting some research of his own. He wanted to learn how all those patients might be able to prevent, arrest, or even reverse their medical problems.

During his study, Esselstyn became convinced that what we eat plays a critical role in our health. He believed that the same superior diet could be employed to fight all chronic diseases, but he needed a good place to start testing his theory. Although his surgery was more related to cancers of the breast and the thyroid, he felt he might be able to prove his theory better by applying it to heart disease. Although not a cardiologist, Esselstyn said, "What better way to treat heart disease than to simply treat its cause?"[27]

So he began a self-funded independent study in his home, with his wife, Ann, in the all-important role of cook. The Cleveland Clinic provided twenty-four high-risk heart patients who could no longer be treated with conventional interventions or had refused further treatment. He told me about raising money himself so that they could purchase angiograms (X-rays) from the clinic. Those X-rays would be needed to illustrate the physical reversal of the heart disease that he expected to see in his patients.

After explaining the dietary guidelines to his patients—which he and his wife also followed—he began to treat these very sick patients with nothing but whole, plant-based foods. Within months, the patients began to improve, and after a few years, the results were outstanding. The seventeen patients who complied with the dietary guidelines had suffered a combined total of forty-nine cardiac events in the eight years leading up to the intervention. In the eleven years after the intervention began, there was not a single cardiac event for the entire group. Since then, Esselstyn has treated hundreds of patients and maintains a near 100 percent success rate for those who comply with the guidelines.[28]

WHOLE, PLANT-BASED FOODS

"Whole, plant-based foods" are the most important words in this entire book. The most nutritious foods are whole plants, still in nature's package. Cooked or raw, a broad combination of these foods is the key to Dr. Esselstyn's heart disease–reversing diet.

Today, Esselstyn is the director of the Cardiovascular Disease Prevention and Reversal Program of the Wellness Institute at the Cleveland

Clinic. He treats hundreds of patients per year. Sadly, hardly any of them are referred by their cardiologist. His patients come to him primarily because of internet searches and word of mouth. Among them are cardiologists and other senior physicians who seek his treatment for themselves and their families but are reluctant to refer their patients. We're optimistic that this phenomenon is temporary, which we discuss further in Chapter 8.

John McDougall, MD. McDougall came to the same conclusions as Esselstyn but arrived at them via a completely different route. After graduating from medical school at Michigan State and interning in Honolulu, McDougall chose to practice on the Big Island of Hawaii. While working with thousands of patients there, he dealt with both recent immigrants from different parts of Asia and some of the third- and fourth-generation Americans from those same Asian countries. McDougall found that many of his patients' problems were chronic diseases like diabetes, cancer, heart disease, and arthritis. He also found that after treating them, as he had been trained, with the conventional pills and procedures, very few of them became healthy. At the same time, he noticed that his first-generation patients—the ones who ate their traditional diets of grains and vegetables—were trim, fit, and not afflicted with chronic diseases. That's how McDougall learned about the power of plant-based nutrition. Inspired by their example, he sought more education in nutrition so that he would someday be able to truly help his patients get healthy.

Reading the scientific literature, McDougall began to fully comprehend the limitations of modern medicine. He soon became convinced that a diet of whole, plant-based foods had the potential to not only prevent chronic disease but also cure it. Like Esselstyn, however, he soon found that this idea was not well received by his colleagues. Despite this resistance, McDougall remains a dedicated physician who is committed to helping his patients regain their health. Besides writing many books on the topic, he has personally treated thousands of patients and reports (in lectures and videos) a remarkable success rate of over 90 percent with patients who suffer from chronic diseases like type 2 diabetes, hypertension, and heart disease.

Dean Ornish, MD. Since receiving his medical training at Baylor College of Medicine, Harvard Medical School, and Massachusetts General Hospital, Ornish has become a giant in the field of medicine. Unlike Esselstyn's treatment, which focuses only on diet, Ornish's program includes stress management techniques and exercise in addition to a vegetarian diet that features "all you can eat" of approved foods, including fruits, vegetables, and grains. In a random trial, including an experimental group and a control group, on average, the total cholesterol levels of the experimental group dropped from 227 mg/dL to 172 mg/dL, and after a year, the frequency, duration, and severity of their chest pain dropped by 91 percent. Meanwhile, the control group, despite the fact that they received the standard care for heart disease, reported that the frequency, duration, and severity of their chest pain got worse. Further, the cholesterol levels and the blockage in their arteries were much worse.[29]

In *The China Study*, Dr. T. Colin Campbell sums up the efforts of Ornish, Esselstyn, and others before them: "Their dietary treatments not only relieve the symptoms of chest pain, but they also treat the cause of heart disease and can eliminate future coronary events. There are no surgical or chemical heart disease treatments, at the Cleveland Clinic or anywhere else, that can compare to these impressive results."[30] Further, these pioneers in the field of heart disease are finally receiving official recognition. In August 2010, for the first time ever, the Centers for Medicare and Medicaid Services announced that Medicare will pay for intensive diet and exercise programs developed under the Ornish and Pritikin brands for reducing cardiovascular event risk. Nathan Pritikin, though not a doctor, developed a diet similar to Ornish's, which reached millions of people after the publication of his best seller, *The Pritikin Program for Diet and Exercise*.

Joel Fuhrman, MD. A former world-class figure skater, second in the U.S. National Pairs Championships in 1973, and a front-runner for the U.S. Olympic team, Fuhrman suffered a severe injury that put him on crutches for over a year and derailed his future skating career—eventually leading him to a career in nutritional medicine. His interest in nutrition, to maximize performance as a skater, led him to undergo a therapeutic fast to aid in his healing. Interestingly, that earlier exposure to the world of superior and therapeutic nutrition played a big role in motivating him to become a physician specializing in nutrition.

Later, during medical school at the University of Pennsylvania, he observed that patients there were treated with conventional procedures and medications, but that they rarely completely regained their health. He saw patients suffer and die needlessly while under the care of modern medicine. Based on his earlier experiences with superior nutrition, he remained convinced that people everywhere could get well if only they were able to leverage the powers of a powerful natural diet.

Joel went on to graduate from the University of Pennsylvania School of Medicine in 1988 and has been practicing nutritional medicine for over twenty years. His best-selling book *Eat to Live* was published in 2003 (Little, Brown) with multiple printings both domestic and abroad. His other six books include *Disease-Proof Your Child*, a book that helped open my son's eyes to the power of health promoting plant-based nutrition—as he wanted to give his four children the best possible chance to enjoy vibrant health for their entire lives.

Dr. Fuhrman's experience and his results in optimizing the therapeutic potential of nutrition are not limited to dramatic weight loss stories, reversal of heart disease and diabetes—but also migraines, asthma, fibromyalgia, and autoimmune diseases. Also, he is actively involved in scientific research in human nutrition, and his discoveries on food addiction and human hunger have changed the scientific landscape regarding hunger and appetite control. His most recent study was published in *Nutrition Journal*, November 2010, entitled, "The Changing Perception of Hunger on a High Nutrient Density Diet."

Neal Barnard, MD. Born and raised in North Dakota, Barnard graduated from the George Washington University School of Medicine in Washington, DC. He founded and remains the president of the Physicians Committee for Responsible Medicine, a nonprofit organization that promotes preventive medicine. He grew up in a cattle-raising family, and his father was also a doctor who spent his entire life treating diabetes. In Barnard's book about reversing diabetes, he chronicles the work that has been done by those before him and also his part in numerous studies at George Washington University.[31]

In 1979, researchers at the University of Kentucky, under the direction of Dr. James Anderson, studied twenty men with type 2 diabetes, which makes up 90 percent of all diabetes cases. High in fiber and carbohydrates, their experimental diet included plenty of vegetables, fruits, whole grains, and beans—a near-vegetarian diet. More than half the men were able to stop taking insulin entirely within just sixteen days.[32] Fifteen years later, a study of 197 men at UCLA showed much the same result, with 140 of them able to stop their medications entirely.[33] Another series of studies began at George Washington University in 1999 and added more evidence to the body of knowledge that type 2 diabetes is reversible with a diet of whole, plant-based foods. All these studies are reviewed in detail in *Dr. Neal Barnard's Program for Reversing Diabetes*.

T. Colin Campbell, PhD. Even before medical doctors Esselstyn, McDougall, Ornish, Fuhrman, and Barnard were making their own discoveries, a future professor of nutritional biochemistry at Cornell University had already begun to uncover what he referred to as some "dark secrets"[34] on the scientific side of the disease debate. Early in his career, after receiving his MS and PhD from Cornell, Campbell worked in research at MIT and later held a faculty position at Virginia Tech in the late 1960s and early 1970s. During that time, he coordinated a USAID-supported program for malnourished young children in the Philippines. The aim of the program was simple: make sure that children were getting as much protein as possible, as it was widely thought that much of the childhood malnutrition in the world was caused by a lack of protein, especially from animal-based foods. Yet, as he reports in his book *The China Study*, he found that the children who ate the highest-protein diets—the children of the wealthiest families—were the ones most likely to get cancer.

FACTS ABOUT T. COLIN CAMPBELL

- He is currently professor emeritus of nutritional biochemistry at Cornell.
- He organized and directed the largest single study of diet, health, and disease in the history of the world, the China-Cornell-Oxford Project.
- In 1975, he returned to Cornell at age forty as a full professor with tenure— a very rare move in academia.
- He has received over seventy grant years of peer-reviewed research funding (mostly from the National Institutes of Health).
- He has authored over 400 scientific research papers during his career.
- At Cornell, he set records in just about every category—fields of study, research, and publications—by raising the most money and receiving the most citations.
- He served on the U.S. Senate Select Committee on Nutrition and Human Needs, chaired by George McGovern.
- He was awarded the coveted Jacob Gould Schurman Endowed Chair at Cornell in 1985 and was the only professor in the Department of Nutritional Sciences so honored.
- When the legendary long-term Cornell president Frank Rhodes retired in 1995, he cited Campbell's China Project in his farewell address to 8,000 people as "one of the greatest embodiments of Cornell excellence to take place during my twenty-two years at the helm of this great institution."[35]

He then noticed a research report from India with some disturbing findings that related to what he had observed in the Philippines. Laboratory studies there showed that increased animal protein in the diet promoted liver cancer in every one of the test animals.

He writes:

> This information countered everything I had been taught. It was heretical to say that protein wasn't healthy, let alone say it promoted cancer. It was a defining moment in my career. Investigating such a provocative question so early in my career was not a very wise choice. Questioning protein and animal-based foods in general ran the risk of my being labeled a heretic, even if it passed the test of "good science."[36]

After his early discovery in the Philippines, Campbell carefully continued his research into the relationship between animal protein and cancer, seeking to understand not only if but also how animal protein might promote cancer. "I was able to study a provocative topic without provoking knee-jerk responses that arise with radical ideas."[37] His well-planned approach led to handsomely funded research for the next twenty-seven years by some of the leading health institutions in the United States: the National Institutes of Health (NIH), the American Cancer Society, and the American Institute for Cancer Research. Through his comprehensive studies, Campbell and his team found more startling information:

- The protein that most consistently and strongly promoted cancer was casein, which makes up 87 percent of cow's milk protein. That's right, cow's milk protein promoted all stages of the cancer process.
- Not all proteins promoted cancer. The safe proteins were derived from plants, including wheat and soy.

Beginning in 1983, Campbell organized and directed an ongoing project responsible for nationwide surveys of diet, lifestyle, and mortality in the People's Republic of China and later in Taiwan. Known as "the China Study," the project eventually produced more than 8,000 statistically significant associations between various dietary factors and disease. Among the key findings:

- People who ate the most animal-based foods had the most chronic diseases.
- Even relatively small amounts of animal-based foods were associated with adverse effects.
- People who ate the most plant-based foods were the healthiest and tended to avoid chronic disease.

Labeling the study the "Grand Prix of epidemiology," a *New York Times* article in May 1990 reported: "Early findings from the most comprehensive large study ever undertaken of the relationship between diet and the risk of developing disease are challenging much of American dietary dogma. The study, being conducted in China, paints a bold portrait of a plant-based eating plan that is more likely to promote health than disease."[38]

As Campbell began discovering some of the "dark secrets" early in his career, many colleagues urged him to keep this information to himself or he would not be able to get more funding, and that would mean the end of his career. But his wife, Karen, insisted that he tell his complete story "for the children of the world."[39] Now widely recognized as the world's leading authority on plant-based nutrition, he has helped to legitimize (with scientific proof) the clinical work of many medical doctors who discovered some of these same remedies on their own.

In *The China Study*, after reviewing the effects of plant-based nutrition on a wide range of chronic diseases, he sums up his conclusion as follows: "When a whole foods, plant-based diet is demonstrably beneficial for such a wide variety of diseases, is it possible that humans were meant to consume any other diet? I say no, and I think you'll agree."[40]

What Is the Optimal Diet for Humans?

The upsurge of knowledge in the field of disease prevention has had wide repercussions. More and more mainstream scientists are recognizing the benefits of a change in diet for their patients. Dr. William C. Roberts, the esteemed editor of the *American Journal of Cardiology*, has pointed out: "[A]lthough we think we are one, and we act as if we are one, human beings are not natural carnivores. When we kill animals to eat them, they end up killing us because their flesh, which contains cholesterol and saturated fat, was never intended for human beings, who are natural herbivores."[41]

Our hands, our teeth, our intestines—our entire bodies—are designed to eat plants. Although our ancestors ate almost anything they could get their hands on, that doesn't mean it was good for them. Nor does it mean they needed the animal protein to become big and strong. In addition to all the essential vitamins, minerals, and phytochemicals, a natural plant diet provides us with the fiber that we need. In his best-selling book *Eat to Live*, Dr. Joel Fuhrman describes the importance of this key nutrient: "When you eat mostly natural plant foods, such as fruits, vegetables, and beans, you get large amounts of various types of fiber . . . The fibers slow down glucose absorption and control the rate of digestion. Plant fibers have complex physiological effects in the digestive tract that offer a variety of benefits, such as lowering cholesterol."[42] Meat, fish, poultry, and all other animal foods contain no fiber; it is found only in plant-based foods.

The American Dietetic Association reports that most of us don't even come close to the recommended intake of twenty grams to thirty-five grams of fiber a day. While thirty-five grams of fiber would be a dramatic improvement for most people eating the typical Western diet, the fiber in a truly health-promoting optimal diet would be more than double that amount. On NutritionData.com, an analysis of a near 100 percent whole-foods, plant-based diet demonstrates that it typically delivers well over seventy grams of fiber per day. I simply added up the fiber in all of my meals of whole plants (fruits, vegetables, legumes, grains, nuts, and seeds) for my typical day. The total always exceeds seventy grams of fiber.

As herbivores, the natural food for our species is plants. We know from a vast amount of research that the healthiest form of plant foods for us is whole and unrefined (fruits, vegetables, grains, legumes, nuts, and seeds). Consumers of the typical Western diet get a paltry 5 percent of their calories from these whole plant foods. The remaining 95 percent of our calories comes from unhealthy foods like meat, added sugar, oil, cheese, chips, sweets, sodas, fries, and other highly refined products with very low amounts of nutrients per calorie.

Some vegetarians and vegans would argue that the optimal diet is 100 percent raw or consists of only fruits and vegetables. They may be right, but the fact is there have not been enough scientific studies to determine the unequivocal optimal diet with conclusive answers to questions like these. How much should be raw? How much should be cooked? How much should be grains, or greens? While the debate about some of these details continues, a growing number of physicians and nutritional scientists educated in some of our leading universities has discovered some common ground on this topic. This common ground is summed up in Dr. Campbell's description of the optimal diet for humans: "[T]here is overwhelming scientific support for one, simple optimal diet—a whole foods, plant-based diet."[43]

Likewise, Dr. Esselstyn's diet allows virtually all whole plant foods, whether cooked or not, and his diet has been successful in reversing advanced heart disease in close to 100 percent of his patients. The bottom line is that people must choose the diet style that works best for them and their family. After learning the not-so-well-known truths about nutrition, each person must choose his own dietary path—one that he can embrace, enjoy, and sustain for the rest of his life. We must remember that even the perfect diet is of no value if we are unable to stick with it.

Promoting Health and Your Ideal Weight

All the experts quoted previously advocate a whole-foods, plant-based diet. Does that mean 100 percent? In nature, the ideal would be 100 percent; however, that may not be practical for many in today's world. Some experts define the optimal diet as one in which at least 80 percent of the calories are derived from whole, unrefined, plant-based foods, with an emphasis on green leafy vegetables, legumes, and fresh fruits. While going halfway and moving up to 40 percent of calories from these highly nutritious foods would definitely be a good move, many experts agree that to have the maximum protection against disease and to enjoy vibrant health your entire life, you really need to shoot for 80 percent or better. That will also ensure that you exceed fifty grams of fiber per day, and that alone will make a huge difference in the way your body functions.

Studies show that most weight-loss diets have a 95 percent failure rate; only 5 percent of the people manage to lose weight and keep it off. So what's the problem? Many diets aimed at weight loss are unsustainable, are lacking in valuable nutrients, and usually require some level of deprivation. With the typical Western diet, no matter how much you eat, your body never gets enough nutrients and is continually craving more food. Of course, all this adds up to a population of overfed and undernourished people.

The simple way to achieve your ideal weight and optimal health is to adopt a permanent diet style based on nutritional excellence. Once you learn how to select, prepare, and eat the right kinds of foods, your body will take care of the rest without calorie counting, portion control, or deprivation. We're talking about a diet style based on maximizing the consumption of whole, unrefined, plant-based foods. How simple is that?

You may be asking, "Will I ever be able to really enjoy eating like I did before?" The short answer is a resounding *yes*. You will very likely come to enjoy your food even more. Your tastes will change once you begin to eat the healthy foods, and you will lose the cravings that you once had for the deadly combination of fat, salt, and sugar. Satisfaction with food goes beyond taste. It also includes a feeling of lightness, energy, and satisfaction that has been missing from our meals for a long time. You won't truly understand or appreciate this point until you treat your body to the optimal diet long enough for it to fully experience the benefits that the diet will provide.

It all sounds rosy, doesn't it? Get out with the gorillas, and have a feast. No doubt, questions have been forming in your mind as you have read this chapter. The medical breakthroughs are fine, but they fly in the face of everything we have been taught about nutrition. What exactly is the story with protein? How could dairy products be bad for you? What about the fact that plants don't contain vitamin D or vitamin B12? Beyond these basic questions, you may also have some more practical ones, like: what would I do at my neighbor's next backyard barbeque? We address all these questions in later chapters. But first, let's explore in more detail the many health-related implications of a whole-foods, plant-based diet.

"Knowledge does not come to us in details, but in flashes of light from heaven."

—Henry David Thoreau, *Life without Principle*

2

YOUR HEALTH AT RISK

"A man too busy to take care of his health is like a mechanic
too busy to take care of his tools."

—Spanish proverb

Almost everyone would put health right up there with family
in terms of what's most important in life. It ranks way ahead
of money, for without health, life isn't much fun, regardless
of how much wealth you have. Given the importance of health, it's
surprising that people don't understand more about what they need to
do to optimize their health.

Many people take their health for granted until they are faced with a
crisis. They believe that bad health is a random event that can happen
to anyone. Usually, their first jolt of their mortality is a heart attack,
a diagnosis of type 2 diabetes, or the advice to have a colonoscopy to
prevent cancer. Millions of people live in fear that a deadly disease
may attack them at any time. In the midst of all this bad news, we
continue to hear about some medical breakthrough or wonder drug
that may solve some problem. Heart surgery and cancer prevention
and treatment have become major industries, and we've witnessed all

sorts of developments in insulin injections. We continue to hold out hope that human ingenuity will create a magic cure. The problem is an analysis of the hard facts would suggest that our many health-related problems are not likely to be resolved anytime soon.

Let's start with the cost of health-care. As mentioned previously, according to Organization for Economic Cooperation and Development (OECD) data gathered in 2009, the cost of health-care in the United States as a percent of GDP has risen steadily from 5.2 percent in 1960 to 16 percent in 2007. During that forty-seven-year period, the cost of health-care as a percent of GDP rose every year. Further, the Congressional Budget Office is predicting that it will double again to 31 percent in the next twenty-five years.[44]

The picture doesn't become brighter when we look at individual diseases. We are not winning the war on cancer. In the past forty years, despite advances in certain types of cancer therapies, overall cancer rates have declined only slightly. Heart disease is still the leading cause of death in the United States, despite the fact that we now understand much more about plaque and blood clots than we used to. Obesity and diabetes are both running rampant, and the risk to children has grown ominously. As ads for osteoporosis, high blood pressure, and erectile dysfunction medications indicate, these diseases are ubiquitous. We are one sick nation, as are other nations who consume a similarly rich diet. In *The China Study*, Dr. Campbell summarizes the state of health in the United States:

- 82 percent of our adults have at least one risk factor for heart disease.
- 81 percent of us take at least one medication during any given week.
- 50 percent of us take at least one prescription drug per week.
- 65 percent of us are overweight.
- 31 percent of us are obese.

- Roughly one in three youths is already overweight or currently at risk.
- About 150 million adults have dangerously high cholesterol levels.
- About 50 million people have high blood pressure.
- Over 63 million people have lower back pain.[45]

Most people have come to the conclusion that these dire statistics are a normal part of aging and that we can't do much to improve our odds. But they are normal only in our *fast-food nation* and only relatively recently. For instance, we tend to assume that heart disease has always plagued people as they get older, but this is not true at all. Dr. John McDougall gives a vivid example: "I worked for a Chinese-trained medical oncologist in 1977 as part of my residency. He told me that when he was a medical student in Hong Kong, heart attacks were so rare that whenever one occurred doctors all over the city rushed to the autopsy lab to see this medical curiosity."[46]

The reason our fights against major diseases are not succeeding is because the advances in modern medicine are attacking the symptoms of the problem, not the root causes. In the last chapter, we saw that medical breakthroughs of a different sort have been made—in the field of nutrition. Buried among the news of fabulous medical break-throughs and miracle drugs is a simpler fact of life: what you put into your body affects how your body functions. The first discoveries in how nutrition affects health were made in the field of heart disease, and these were rapidly succeeded by medical studies that related the role of animal protein and fat to a wide spectrum of other modern plagues, such as diabetes, cancer, and osteoporosis. Let's look at each of these major diseases and find out how their grim progression has been stopped and even reversed by a simple change in diet.

Mud in the Pump

The first symptom many victims of heart disease experience is a heart attack. Since the first attack doesn't strike most people until they are fifty or older, we naturally assume that the disease is associated with aging. And there's nothing we can do about it, right? Wrong on both counts![47]

Heart disease is directly related to restricted blood flow as a result of the buildup of plaque in our arteries. Plaque is a semihardened accumulation of substances, notably cholesterol, which lines the inner walls of blood vessels. Research has shown that the growth of plaque is the natural result of eating our rich Western diet. Studies have shown that rather than developing during middle age, when people tend to exercise less, plaque buildup begins early in life. Autopsies of fallen U.S. soldiers in Korea, for instance, revealed that almost 80 percent of these young men had advanced heart disease. In contrast, the arteries of the plant-eating Korean soldiers were largely clean, free of fatty deposits.[48] In June 2008, *USA Today* reported the following alarming statistics from the National Health and Nutrition Examination Survey conducted from 1999 to 2004. These are the percentages of Americans, by age group, that have cardiovascular disease:

- 11 percent for ages 20 to 39
- 39 percent for ages 40 to 59
- 73 percent for ages 60 to 79
- 88 percent for ages 80 and older[49]

According to these numbers, almost 90 percent of the people over eighty have some form of artery disease—not simply because they're old but because they've been consuming a meat-based diet for sixty years longer than the young adults.

Despite the incredible amounts of money spent on heart disease, the situation has not improved. Dr. Campbell points out in *The China Study*:

[T]he incidence rate (not death rate) for heart disease is about the same as it was in the early 1970s. In other words, while we don't die as much from heart disease, we still get it as often as we used to. It seems that we simply have gotten slightly better at postponing death from heart disease, but *we have done nothing to stop the rate at which our hearts become diseased.*[50]

The link between fat and heart disease was established by scientific research long ago. The granddaddy of this research is the Framingham Heart Study, named after a Boston suburb where the tests were conducted. Starting in 1948, scientists studied 5,209 Framingham men and women between the ages of thirty and sixty for a period of twenty years. Their findings led to a revolution in thinking about risk factors such as high blood pressure, cigarette smoking, and especially blood cholesterol levels. Many of their findings have become the basis of how scientists measure heart disease. To give an idea of its widespread influence, more than 1,000 scientific papers have been published from this study.[51]

Dr. Dean Ornish, famous for his diet that reverses heart disease, wrote about the misconceptions that many people have about what is healthy. He explains that the "normal" ranges of the past were obtained by taking a sample of everyone's cholesterol and finding that the majority of Americans had total cholesterol levels well above 200. He points out that those numbers were *average*, not necessarily *normal*. He uses the Framingham Study to explain normal: "No one in the Framingham Study has had a heart attack whose blood cholesterol level has remained consistently under 150. In countries where heart disease is very rare, blood cholesterol levels remain at about this level. Thus, a normal cholesterol level is around 150 or less.[52]

Dr. Ornish goes on to show just how dangerous elevated blood cholesterol levels can be. He cites a study led by Dr. Jeremiah Stamler at Northwestern University, in which Stamler and his colleagues studied over 350,000 men who were thirty-five to fifty-seven years old.

They found that men whose blood cholesterol levels were above 180 had an increased mortality from heart disease. Over a six-year period, cholesterol readings between 182 and 202 increased the mortality rate by 29 percent; levels between 203 and 220 increased the rate by 73 percent; levels of 221 to 244 raised it by 121 percent; and levels of 245 or above increased it by 242 percent.[53]

If the "normal" level in the United States is over 200, is it any wonder that so many people have heart attacks?

The medical community has addressed the problem mainly through surgery and drugs. While invasive interventions have helped some people, the shocking fact is how little they have helped others. Dr. Campbell reports the sobering facts about heart bypass surgery:

The most pronounced benefit of this procedure is relief of angina, or chest pain. About 70–80% of patients who undergo bypass surgery remain free of this crippling chest pain for one year. *But this benefit doesn't last.* Within three years of the operation, up to one-third of patients will suffer from chest pain again. Within ten years half of the bypass patients will have died, had a heart attack or had their chest pain return.[54]

The good news is that this sinister disease can be prevented and even reversed at almost any age. Dr. Caldwell B. Esselstyn says in all his speeches, "Heart disease is a toothless paper tiger that need never exist; and if it does exist, it need never progress." We discussed in Chapter 1 how Dr. Esselstyn successfully reversed advanced heart disease in all seventeen of his Cleveland Clinic patients who complied with his guidelines to eat a diet rich in fruits, vegetables, and other whole plant foods. Similar results have been reported by Drs. Ornish, Fuhrman, and McDougall, proving beyond a doubt that heart disease is reversible with a health-promoting, whole-foods, plant-based diet. Of the millions of heart attacks that occur around the globe each year, Dr. Fuhrman says:

[E]very single one of those heart attacks is a terrible tragedy, as it could have been avoided. So many people die needlessly because of wrong, weak, and practically worthless information from the government, physicians, dietitians, and even health authorities like the American Heart Association. Conventional guidelines are simply insufficient to offer real protection for those wanting to protect themselves from heart disease.[55]

Dr. Neal Barnard shows one effect of the misinformation that spreads among the general public. Most people believe that switching from red meat to chicken or fish will help prevent heart attacks. However, Dr. Barnard says:

In studies, chicken-and-fish diets are routinely disappointing. When researchers test diets that include even modest amounts of chicken and fish for their effect on cholesterol, they find that these foods reduce "bad" low-density lipoprotein (LDL) cholesterol by only about 5 percent compared to an unrestricted diet. LDL cholesterol is the kind that increases the risk of heart problems. Much more effective are diets that eliminate animal products altogether. Our most recent study using this sort of diet cut LDL cholesterol by more than 20 percent. That's four times better than the chicken-and-fish approach.[56]

In a paper published in the September 2010 *American Journal of Cardiology*, Dr. Esselstyn describes the futility of the current method of treating heart disease. He says the interventions and pharmaceutical treatments are only a stopgap treatment, that they're doing nothing to address the causative factors. He cites four separate plant-eating cultures around the world in which coronary disease is virtually nonexistent and then makes a telling point about what happened when the diet of a group of Europeans was altered by decree. Deaths from heart disease and stroke plummeted from 1939 to 1945 in Norway during World War II, when the occupying German forces deprived the Norwegians of their livestock, forcing a rationing that greatly diminished their animal-based foods. But after the hostilities ceased and the normal consumption of meat and dairy was restored in 1945, death rates from stroke and heart attack approached their pre-1945 levels.[57]

Studies such as this have been conducted so many times that the link between animal foods and heart disease is becoming common knowledge. The same word is getting out about the link between animal foods and diabetes. Yet while heart disease has leveled off—at its astronomically high level—diabetes is exploding into a worldwide crisis all its own.

ERECTILE DYSFUNCTION CAN SAVE YOUR LIFE

You've seen the ads a numbing number of times. *When the moment is right, will you be ready?* Rather than taking a little blue pill, though, men should know a simple biological fact of life. As Dr. Esselstyn points out, the cause of heart disease and erectile dysfunction is essentially the same: restricted blood flow as a result of the buildup of plaque in our arteries.[58] Neither disease is the natural result of aging but rather the natural result of eating the rich Western diet for many years. So if you're lucky enough to have erectile dysfunction before your first heart attack, let it be your wake-up call to take action *now*.

Sugar Gone Sour

The numbers for diabetes are really getting scary. One in twelve people in the United States is diabetic, and the incidence of the disease is increasing rapidly, rising 33 percent from 1990 to 1998.[59] In addition, one-third of the people who have diabetes don't even know that they have it. There are an estimated 800,000 diabetics in New York City alone, a staggering one in every eight adults. City officials are now describing the problem as a bona fide epidemic.[60]

Diabetes is a chronic disorder caused by the body's inability to process glucose, or blood sugar, because of a lack of insulin, a hormone produced in the pancreas that allows the body to use and store glucose. Dr. Campbell provides a useful guide to the process:

Normal metabolism goes like this:

- We eat food.
- The food is digested and the carbohydrate part is broken down into simple sugars, much of which is glucose.
- Glucose (blood sugar) enters the blood, and insulin is produced by the pancreas to manage its transport and distribution around the body.
- Insulin, acting like an usher, opens doors for glucose into different cells for a variety of purposes. Some of the glucose is converted to short-term energy for immediate cell use, and some is stored as long-term energy (fat) for later use.[61]

Diabetics cannot produce enough insulin to convert glucose properly. This causes the blood sugar to rise to dangerous levels.

Over 90 percent of diabetes cases are type 2, formerly referred to as "adult-onset diabetes." But because up to 45 percent of the new cases in children are type 2, the age-specific label has been dropped. A 2006 *New York Times* article on diabetes began with this sad situation in a New York City hospital:

Begin on the sixth floor, third room from the end, swathed in fluorescence: a 60-year-old woman was having two toes sawed off. One floor up, corner room: a middle-aged man sprawled, recuperating from a kidney transplant. Next door: nerve damage. Eighth floor, first room to the left: stroke. Two doors down: more toes being removed. Next room: a flawed heart.

As always, the beds at Montefiore Medical Center in the Bronx were filled with a universe of afflictions. In truth, these assorted burdens were all the work of a single illness: diabetes. Room after room, floor after floor, diabetes. On any given day, hospital officials say, nearly half the patients are there for some trouble precipitated by the disease.[62]

In spite of its powerful rise in recent years, there is some good news. With the right diet, type 2 diabetes can be reversed completely in over 90 percent of the cases, and type 1 diabetics can significantly lower their insulin dosage.[63] Dr. Barnard candidly discusses the standard treatment regimen for type 2 diabetes prescribed by most medical teams: "For most people, this sort of diet change has only a very limited effect. Weight loss is generally modest, and the diet alone typically is not enough to bring blood sugar under control. Sooner or later, you and your doctor are likely to decide that the 'diabetes diet' is not helping very much, and your doctor will add various drugs."[64]

He goes on to say that certain recommendations don't make much sense. In other parts of the world, no one would follow, for instance, the advice not to eat carbohydrates.

Large population studies showed that diabetes was rare in Japan, China, Thailand, and other Asian countries. It was similarly rare in parts of Africa. These studies also showed something else: People in countries where diabetes was uncommon were not following anything like a "diabetes diet." They did not avoid carbohydrates; they ate starchy foods every day. In Asia and Africa, rice and other grains, starchy vegetables, bean dishes, and noodles are staples.[65]

Dr. Ornish points out how Western eaters can make a simple change to achieve the same results. "The bran and fiber in whole wheat flour and brown rice prevent an excessive insulin response. Thus, you don't have to give up pasta, bread, or rice; just change to whole wheat pasta, whole wheat bread, and brown rice."[66]

Fortunately, the same powerful diet that reverses heart disease can reverse type 2 diabetes. Thousands of people have completely eliminated their type 2 diabetes while following the whole foods, plant-based treatment regimen, as practiced by Joel Fuhrman, John McDougall, and Dean Ornish. Dr. Fuhrman sums up his feelings on the disease in *Eat to Live*: "Patients are told to learn to live with their diabetes and to learn to control it because it can't be cured. 'No, no, and no!' I say. 'Don't live with it, get thin and get rid of it.'"[67]

How can a plant-based diet have such an effect on diabetes? Dr. Ornish explains how such foods work inside your body:

> Complex carbohydrates include fruits, vegetables, grains, and legumes (beans) in their natural forms . . . [The] sugars found in complex carbohydrates are absorbed slowly, thereby helping to keep blood sugar levels constant and so they do not stimulate your body to produce excess amounts of insulin. In contrast, simple carbohydrates—sugar and other concentrated sweeteners like high fructose corn syrup and honey, and alcohol, which your body converts to sugar—are absorbed rapidly, causing your blood sugar to rapidly increase. In response, your body secretes insulin to lower blood sugar levels to normal.[68]

The key point to gain is that you can control how your body works. When you eat a diet that doesn't cause your blood sugar to bounce up and down like a yo-yo, you don't need outside intervention—like an insulin injection—to regulate your metabolism. Your body moves in rhythm with the food you eat.

The Big C

Cancer is the most insidious, dreaded disease of our time. Almost everyone knows a loved one or a friend who has heard the chilling diagnosis and the awful range of life expectancy and has undergone the nauseating rounds of radiation, chemotherapy, and/or surgery. Volumes upon volumes have been written about the wide array of cancers and their treatment since Richard Nixon declared war on cancer in 1971. Yet for all the billions of dollars spent on its study, only limited advances have been made with certain types of cancer. Forty years later, for most people it is still a death sentence. Dr. Campbell states, "If you are male in this country, the American Cancer Society says that you have a 47% chance of getting cancer. If you are female, you fare a little better, but you still have a whopping 38% lifetime chance of getting cancer."[69] Not only is cancer devastating on a personal level; according to a Huffington Post article in August 2010, "Cancer is the world's top 'economic killer' as well as its likely leading cause of death, the American Cancer Society contends in a new report it will present at a global cancer conference in China this week . . . Cancer's economic toll was $895 billion in 2008—equivalent to 1.5 percent of the world's gross domestic product."[70]

The links between diet and various forms of cancer have been established in many studies. As just one example, a 2007 report of the World Cancer Research Fund International includes an extensive overview of hundreds of studies that found links between obesity and a wide range of cancers. The report says:

> The evidence that greater body fatness is a cause of cancers of the esophagus (adenocarcinoma), pancreas, colorectum, breast (postmenopause), endometrium, and kidney is convincing. Greater body fatness is probably a cause of gallbladder cancer, both directly and indirectly through the formation of gallstones. There is also limited evidence suggesting that greater body fatness is a cause of liver cancer. The evidence that abdominal fatness is a cause of colorectal cancer is convincing, and abdominal fatness is probably a cause of cancers of the pancreas, breast (postmenopause), and endometrium.[71]

It is widely understood that for cancer to occur, the following elements must be in place: a gene, a carcinogen, and the proper chemical environment. It turns out that all cancers share certain characteristics, and there is growing evidence that many of them can be prevented, if not reversed, with dietary intervention.

Dr. Fuhrman states in *Eat to Live*, "Animal-product consumption in general is proportionally associated with multiple types of cancer. A massive international study that amassed data from fifty-nine different countries showed that men who ate the most meat, poultry, and dairy products were the most likely to die from prostate cancer, while those that ate the most unrefined plant foods and nuts were the least likely to succumb to this disease."[72] He cites another study in Germany that found that colon and rectal cancer decreased by 50 percent in adult vegetarians, noting that the protection is greater the longer one consumes a plant-based diet.

The foremost expert on the link between animal protein and cancer is Dr. Campbell. One of the primary subjects of his massive twenty-seven-year China Project was cancer. That's because much of his career has been concentrated on the study of cancer, and he has extensive laboratory experience in several cancers, including those of the liver, breast, and pancreas. His impressive data from the China Project suggest that the ability of diet to slow, stop, or even reverse cancer applies to all cancers. He says there is enough evidence now that:

- Doctors should be discussing the option of using dietary change as a potential path to cancer prevention and treatment.
- The U.S. government should be discussing the idea that the toxicity of our diet is the single biggest cause of cancer.
- Local cancer alliances and institutions should be discussing the possibility of providing information to Americans everywhere on how a whole-foods, plant-based diet may be an incredibly effective anticancer medicine.[73]

Dr. Campbell's research has shown that cancer develops in three stages: initiation, promotion, and progression. The initiation may take only minutes, while the promotion can take decades. By then it may be too late, as the final stage (progression) may take only a few years before the patient dies. A primary culprit that aids in promotion, he discovered, is casein, a nutrient that constitutes 87 percent of the proteins in cow's milk.[74] In the Western world, we have been led to believe that prevention means screening for cancers and then treating them with chemo, surgery, and radiation before it is too late. This is not prevention at all; this is simply "early detection." But what does "early" mean? The problem is that most cancers cannot be detected for decades after their initiation.

Dr. Campbell summarizes: "There is enough evidence now that doctors should be discussing the option of pursuing dietary change as a potential path to cancer prevention and treatment. There is enough evidence now that the U.S. government should be discussing the idea that the toxicity of our diet is the single biggest cause of cancer."[75]

Got Osteoporosis?

You may have first heard about osteoporosis from television ads. Perhaps you have seen the one for Boniva, in which Sally Field talks about not getting enough calcium from such foods as yogurt, spinach, and cheese. Little does she know that two out of three of those calcium-rich foods are doing much more harm than good. It is truly incredible that the very advice given by the dairy industry to control osteoporosis (drink more milk) has actually been shown by studies to aid in the promotion of the disease. Americans consume more cow's milk and its products per person than almost every other population in the world. So Americans should have extremely strong bones, right? Unfortunately, we don't. A study published in 2000 shows that American women age fifty and older have one of the highest rates of hip fractures in the world. The only countries with higher rates are Australia, New Zealand, and some countries in Europe, where people consume even more milk than people in the United States.[76] How is this happening?

Researchers have found that animal protein, unlike plant protein, increases the acid load in the body. The body responds by fighting this unnaturally acidic environment. To neutralize the acid, the body uses calcium, which acts as a base. This calcium is pulled from the bones, and the calcium loss weakens them, putting them at greater risk for fracture.[77]

This startling fact bears repeating. Science has shown that drinking cow's milk and consuming other dairy products is one of the leading causes of osteoporosis. In countries where the percent of calories from animal-based foods approaches zero, this and other chronic diseases are almost completely unknown.

Dr. McDougall cites studies of two different populations that suggest that the higher the level of animal protein intake, the higher the rate of osteoporosis:

- Members of the Bantu tribe living in Africa on low-protein vegetable diets are essentially free of osteoporosis. Genetic relatives of the Bantu in the United States consume plenty of meat and dairy and have osteoporosis nearly as commonly as white people in the United States.
- Eskimos consume a diet very high in animal protein from fish and very high in calcium from the fish bones, yet these very physically active people have one of the highest rates of osteoporosis in the world.[78]

As with heart disease, diabetes, and cancer, there is no lack of information on what causes osteoporosis. It's hardly news that would comfort the American Dairy Association, one of the largest special interest groups in the United States. In Chapter 8, we explore more of the barriers that scientists face in getting out the word about their findings. For now, you should be aware that the link between nutrition and all of these diseases is not based on some isolated study of a mouse population of ten. These studies can be found in numerous medical journals and all over the internet.

But What's in It for Me—Now?

In addition to the many physical benefits of enjoying vibrant health at any age, there is also the matter of dollars and cents. As you move toward a whole-foods, plant-based diet, there will likely be changes in your body that will begin to save you some money. We're talking about fewer trips to the doctor, numerous procedures that you may never need, fewer illnesses requiring treatment, and fewer routine medications that most Westerners take for their entire lives. In addition, the food itself will cost less money. By eliminating meat, dairy, and eggs from your shopping list, you'll likely lower your total grocery bill. You are also likely to find that the healthy meals you order in restaurants cost about half as much as the meat-based entrées. Saving money while getting healthier—not a bad combination.

Conveniently, the same simple diet is good for preventing all diseases and also for promoting vibrant health. When Dr. Campbell was interviewing potential publishers for *The China Study*, one editor asked about possible different diets for different diseases: "'Can you make specific diet plans for each disease, so that every chapter doesn't have the same recommendations?' In other words, could I tell people to eat a specific way for heart disease and a different way for diabetes? The implication, of course, was that the same eating plan for multiple diseases simply wasn't catchy enough, wasn't sufficiently 'marketable.'"[79] Dr. Campbell didn't apologize for the fact that his simple prescription wasn't catchy enough for the editor. Even though it might not promote his book sales, he looked at his simple dietary recommendations as an opportunity to clear away much of the public confusion. Summing it up, he states, "Quite simply, you can maximize health for diseases across the board with one simple diet."[80]

The switch toward consuming more plant-based foods does not have to be an ordeal. You will not end up looking like an Ethiopian refugee after a month. Dr. Barnard received positive comments about his plant-based diet regimen, which is designed for diabetics:

> Setting aside animal products and keeping oily foods to a minimum may sound challenging, but our participants commonly reported just the opposite. One man, Walter, said, "I'm amazed at how easy it was to adapt to this diet. And I feel great. Within 2 months, I lost 20 pounds. And the more amazing thing to me is that my glucose averages have fallen by 30 to 40 points." . . .
>
> Nancy agreed. She felt totally adjusted to the diet within about 30 days. "And within five months of making the change," she said, "my blood sugar fell so much that I was able to stop one of my medications. I have much more energy and really feel tremendous."[81]

Another advantage of a plant-based diet is that you don't have to starve to lose weight. The self-destructive diets like the Atkins Diet and the South Beach Diet can't work over the long term, because you're denying your body the sustenance it needs to live. The fact is, as any qualified nutritionist can tell you, the type of food you eat is more important than the amount you eat. In a study by Harvard Medical School, "investigators studied 141 women, ages thirty-four to fifty-nine. There was virtually no correlation between calorie intake and body weight, even after adjusting for age, physical activity, alcohol, and smoking. The degree of excess weight was linked to fat consumption (especially saturated fat), *independent of calorie intake*."[82]

A lot of folks out there are just not that concerned about what diseases may strike them later in life. But many of those people might be very interested to know what benefits of healthy eating they can start enjoying right away. The experts referenced in these first two chapters have all written about these benefits, and anyone who has ever switched over to a whole-foods, plant-based diet has almost certainly experienced them. The benefits are encompassed in vibrant health—the condition that exists when all 100 trillion of your body's cells are getting all the nutrients they need, along with fresh air and water and the appropriate amount of exercise, sleep, and sunlight. Dr. Campbell reviews the enormous benefits of a healthy lifestyle and includes among them weight loss, more energy, looking and feeling younger, alleviation of constipation, less money spent on prescription drugs, preservation of eyesight, and many others.[83]

Recently, I asked several friends what type of benefits they had experienced since beginning their healthy-eating regimen. Lisa, a thirty-six-year-old teacher and triathlete, reports faster healing, almost no need for deodorant, no cramping during her monthly period, and effortless weight loss (she went from size 8 to size 2 in the first six months). Her eight-year-old son, Andrew, never gets sick anymore and is now able to outrun older kids who were once faster than he was.

A thirty-seven-year-old business executive and personal trainer, Jason, reports better eyesight, sounder sleeping with more dreams, quicker recovery from workouts, and a complete elimination of his decade-long dependence on prescription medication for depression.

Shawn, a twenty-seven-year-old, had no health or weight problems before changing his diet. While a PhD student at Georgia Tech, he learned about the health-promoting diet from his uncle, read one book over a weekend, and completely adopted the diet in less than a month. Shawn reports the following benefits of his change in diet:

- He dropped twenty pounds in the first two weeks.
- He made gains in the weight room at the same time.
- He is rarely thirsty and not usually hungry.
- If he gets sick, it lasts for about twelve hours (instead of days or weeks).
- He now notices the delicate and delicious flavors of plant foods.

- His bowel movements are quick and easy and happen two to three times per day.
- He can now eat as much as he likes without worrying about "dieting."
- He never has to worry about animal-borne food poisoning.
- His fridge never stinks of old milk, cheese, or meat.

He says, "Maybe the most interesting effect is that I feel 'lighter'— sort of like having a clear sinus as opposed to being stuffed up, but for the whole body. It's very refreshing."

Then, there is Nigel, a seventy-two-year-old business consultant and former marathoner. A native of England, he has lived in the United States for over forty years and consumed the typical Western diet from birth until the age of sixty-six. Fortunately, about that time, he saw Joel Fuhrman's book *Eat to Live*, favorably reviewed in both the *New York Times* and the *Economist*. He immediately purchased a copy, adopted the plant-based lifestyle, and has been enjoying vibrant health ever since. Nigel reports the following positive results:

- His blood pressure, cholesterol, and pulse all went down. His total cholesterol is now at 171 with no medications, and his pulse is at 53.
- His medical and food costs are down.
- He takes no supplements or medications of any kind and remains healthy.
- Before he improved his diet, the Red Cross refused to accept his blood because of low iron; now his iron levels are right where they're supposed to be.
- His dentist keeps telling him he wants to use Nigel as an example of how someone his age should take care of himself.
- He doesn't seem to have any ailments: he says his "guts work well," he never gets stomachaches or headaches, and his skin condition and color are also good.

Nigel explains, "Exercise may have something to do with it, but I exercised back when I ate meat. So I attribute the improvements to simple and nutritious eating. I have two older brothers and one younger sister, all of whom are crazy carnivores and all of whom have suffered from serious chronic illnesses—one brother with Parkinson's, the other with heart disease, and sister with breast cancer. No bad signs for me so far."

Fifty-two-year-old Bob has been almost vegan since 2007. His numbers tell the story of his success:

- His weight dropped from 183 to 155 pounds.
- His total cholesterol went from 176 to 124.
- His LDL cholesterol went from 106 to 71.
- His HDL cholesterol went from 37 to 40.
- His triglycerides dropped from 166 to 65.

According to his doctor, he has the same blood chemistry as he did when he was a teenager. His good habits rubbed off on his sons, ages twelve and sixteen, who are now requesting more vegetarian meals and report the following changes:

- Fewer headaches
- Much less acne
- Improved cognitive abilities, fewer mood swings, and happier moods
- Fewer colds
- More energy and no drowsiness after big meals

The bottom line is that by simply eating the natural diet for our species, we all have the power to take charge of our own health, avoid or possibly reverse chronic disease, and enjoy vibrant health for however long we might live. Maybe it's time for us to realize that the way modern medicine is handling our "health-care" is simply not working.

Maybe it's time to think about a completely new way to promote our health, improve our quality of life, and tame this health-care monster once and for all. In the 2010 documentary *Forks over Knives*, Dr. Campbell and Dr. Esselstyn refer to the "nutritionally avoidable" and the "food-borne" diseases and estimate that 70 to 80 percent of the costs of our health-care system could simply be eliminated if everyone shifted to a whole-foods, plant-based diet.[84]

John Robbins, author of *Healthy at 100*, offers a holistic view of how to maintain health and live a happy and active life to a ripe old age. His emphasis is more on "health span" than chronological life span. After an in-depth review of four of the world's healthiest and longest-lived peoples, he discusses the health-promoting diet that they all share. Their vibrant health can be achieved by almost anyone who takes the steps to do so. For most people, the period of great health ends by the time they are in their fifties or sixties. But with proper nutrition, exercise, and motivation, there is no reason that you should not enjoy vibrant health for your entire life—well into your nineties and maybe even to one hundred.

In summary, the current health epidemic in the United States is the normal result of having 300 million people consuming a so-called "balanced diet" that is actually a fat-laden recipe for disaster and nowhere near the natural diet for our species. The toll of chronic diseases on our older citizens is such that the average twenty-first-century American will spend more years caring for parents than for children.

What Are We Passing Down to Our Children?

One of the most important benefits of adopting the whole-foods, plant-based diet is the twofold gift that we can give our children. First, we provide them with a simple road map for how to promote their own heath and that of their children for the rest of their lives. What gift could be more precious than that? Second, we relieve them of the painful and expensive task of caring for their parents—a burden that will consume the lives of so many millions of young people as they support aged, sick, and depressed parents who are being kept alive by the "wonders" of modern medicine.

Do your children a favor: take steps now to prevent the onset of chronic disease for yourself, simultaneously teaching them how to do the same thing for themselves and their children. There is simply nothing more important for you to do as a parent.

In addition to teaching children how to promote their own health, we can all work together to prevent saddling the next generation with the unsustainable cost of health-care that we are currently experiencing. Our overall health-care system, particularly in the United States, is completely unsound, and it's not very likely that the politicians will be able to fix it. The following numbers, as of 2010, summarize the grim situation.

- The *New York Times* reports that the cost of an average family policy is now $13,770.[85] The Congressional Budget Office projects that health-care in the United States will hit 31 percent of the GDP in 2035—up from 5.2 percent in 1960 and 16.1 percent in 2007 (as reported in the Introduction).
- Even as costs go up, the out-of-pocket cost for the worker is going up even faster. The *New York Times* reports that the worker's share of the average policy went up 14 percent compared to only a 3 percent increase in the cost of the policy.[86]
- The *Washington Post* reports the new census numbers indicating that 44 million Americans are now living below the poverty line—the largest number since tracking began fifty-one years ago.[87]
- More than 51 million Americans lack health insurance, the census reported, and a greater-than-ever percentage of those who do have insurance are getting it from the government.[88]

The health-care problem is not going to be resolved by lawmakers arguing over government programs. Whether you are a Democrat or Republican, liberal or conservative, the ultimate solution is a whole new way of looking at the promotion of health throughout the world. The solution is refreshingly simple, and it's right under our noses: it's all about what we put in our mouths every single meal.

"When health is absent, wisdom cannot reveal itself, art cannot become manifest, strength cannot be exerted, wealth is useless and reason is powerless."

—Herophilus, 300 BC

3

WHY NOT PLANT-BASED?

"Loyalty to a petrified opinion never yet broke a chain or freed a human soul."

—Mark Twain

Thirty years ago, my younger brother informed me that he had become a vegetarian. Thinking that he had lost his mind, I wanted to know what was behind such a ludicrous decision. Was it for the love of animals, some hippie fad, or just a twisted desire on his part to be different? I remember asking him all sorts of questions. Where did he get his protein? Did he still eat fish, cheese, and other animal products that weren't as bad as red meat? It was hard for me to accept the fact that my very own brother was doing something as weird as becoming a vegetarian. Next, he would grow long hair, pierce his ears, wear funny shoes, and smoke dope. At that time in my life, weird and vegetarian were synonymous. Looking for some chink in his armor, I was delighted when I discovered that he would still eat meat if someone else was paying for it; hence, I started calling him a freebie-tarian.

While public acceptance of vegetarians has come a long way since 1980, many people still feel that eating vegetables is for weirdos and sissies. Today, just 3.2 percent of Americans consider themselves vege-tarian and only 0.5 percent eschew all animal-based foods and become vegan.[89] For the United Kingdom, the percentage of vegetarians was estimated at 5.6 percent in 2006—much higher than in the United States, possibly because of the higher risk of mad cow disease in the United Kingdom. The prejudice continues despite the growing number of high-profile people who have embraced the vegetable-eating life-style: pro golfer Gary Player, track stars Carl Lewis and Edwin Moses, tennis great Martina Navratilova, Ironman Dave Scott, and NFL all-pro tight end Tony Gonzalez. Even Chelsea Clinton served mostly vegan food at her recent wedding.

The "vegetarians are weird" sentiment represents one of the most common arguments against switching to a health-promoting, whole-foods, plant-based diet. Ironically, many vegetarians are not eating a very healthy diet. They became vegetarians for ethical reasons without fully understanding the health-promoting part of the diet. To promote health, a person needs to maximize his or her consumption of whole plants—in nature's package. Simply avoiding animal-based foods does not consti-tute a healthy diet. As stated previously, those "v" words tell people only what you *don't* eat, but what you *do* eat is far more important.

From a purely nutritional standpoint, animal foods are not needed to maintain good health. But many people have trouble believing this because of common misunderstandings. What about protein? What about calcium? What about vitamin D? What about vitamin B12? What about omega-3 fatty acids? Aren't they antioxidants? Also, everybody knows that plants are sprayed with pesticides. How can that be good for you?

Rather than counter with some vague whole-earth comment like "It's nature's way," let's take a look at the cold, hard scientific facts. Any advice about eating healthy has to cover every single aspect of eating healthy. Otherwise, you're just being sold another bill of goods, and in this modern age of industrial food, that's a problem people face all too often. Here are the most common misconceptions one by one.

Animal Products Are the Best (or Only) Source of Protein

Let's begin with the health argument that you have probably heard the most: "If you don't eat animal products, where do you get your protein?" This argument is twofold:

- You need to eat some animal products to get the protein that you need.
- If you get protein from only plants, you must combine various plants to get all eight of the essential amino acids.

For most people, protein and meat are synonymous; the idea that plants contain sufficient protein is completely foreign. What they don't realize is that all fruits, vegetables, legumes, grains, nuts, and seeds have protein in them (see Table 3.1 for both plant and animal sources of protein). Some of them, such as beans, nuts, broccoli, and spinach, have more than others. We never have to be concerned about getting enough of any of the three macronutrients that contain calories (protein, carbohydrates, and fat) if we simply eat a variety of whole, plant-based foods every day. The beauty of this diet is that it is the natural diet for our species, and nature has packaged everything in these healthy foods in just the right quantities.

Table 3.1 Plant and Animal Foods Containing Protein[90]

A Sampling of Protein-Rich Foods	Percentage of Calories from Protein
Spinach	49
Eggs	33
Watercress	46
Yogurt	19

A Sampling of Protein-Rich Foods	Percentage of Calories from Protein
Zucchini	28
Turkey	41
Broccoli	45
Swiss cheese	30
Asparagus	38
T-bone steak	16

One reason for the misunderstanding is a lack of knowledge of how the body digests protein. Dr. Dean Ornish provides a concise explanation:

Protein is formed from building blocks called amino acids . . . The amino acids that come from plant foods are exactly the same as the amino acids that come from animal foods. When you eat protein, whether from a T-bone steak or from a meal of rice and beans, that protein is digested into the individual amino acid building blocks . . . In other words, the protein that comes from eating a T-bone steak is exactly the same quality as the protein that comes from a meal of rice and beans.[91]

Another reason is that we believe we need to eat far more protein than we really do need. Dr. Ornish estimates that most people eat twice as much protein as they should.[92] Dr. Caldwell Esselstyn makes the same point in his book: "Typically, the Western diet contains an excess of protein—especially animal protein. The nutrition plan that I recommend provides a variety of healthy plant proteins, somewhere between 50 and 70 grams every day. That is entirely adequate for a healthy lifestyle."[93]

Why is too much protein a problem? At least in the case of animal protein, an excess contributes to many health problems, as we discussed in Chapter 2. Dr. John McDougall explains further:

Everyone knows that we need protein and that meat, dairy products, and eggs are concentrated protein sources. Few people know that recommendations to eat these excessive and harmful sources of protein are based on research dealing largely with rats, which at birth need ten times the amount of protein that a human baby does. How many people hear the real protein story, which reveals that the average person living in a modern society consumes enough excess protein every day to cause a mineral imbalance? Animal protein actually washes calcium from the body into the kidney system, leaving calcium-deficient bones and an increased risk of kidney stones.[94]

Addressing the argument that vegetarians need to carefully balance what they eat, Dr. Neal Barnard assures his readers that they will get the full array of proteins they need:

In years past, some nutritionists believed that vegetarians needed to carefully combine various foods in order to get adequate protein. The idea was that foods from plants might be missing one or more amino acids, so only combining foods in certain ways could ensure that you got them all. This notion was set aside long ago. The American Dietetic Association's official position statements make it clear that plant-based diets provide plenty of protein without combining foods in any particular way.[95]

Dr. Joel Fuhrman agrees with this assessment. He has been curing many forms of chronic disease in his patients for over twenty years. In *Eat to Live*, he weighs in on the question of variety:

[Y]ou do not have to be a nutritional scientist or dietitian to figure out what to eat and you don't have to mix and match foods to achieve protein completeness. Any combination of natural foods will supply you with adequate protein, including all eight essential amino acids as well as unessential amino acids . . . It is only when a vegetarian diet revolves around white bread and other processed foods that the protein content falls to low levels. However, the minute you include unprocessed foods such as vegetables, whole grains, beans, or nuts, the diet becomes protein-rich.[96]

Dr. T. Colin Campbell approaches the topic from the scientific viewpoint: "[T]here is a mountain of compelling research showing that . . . plant protein, which allows for slow but steady synthesis of new proteins, is the healthiest type of protein."[97] People have been led to believe that they must meticulously combine proteins from different plant sources during each meal so that they can mutually compensate for each other's amino acid deficits. Like the other experts, Dr. Campbell disagrees that there's a need for combining proteins: "We now know that through enormously complex metabolic systems, the human body can derive all the essential amino acids from the natural variety of plant proteins that we encounter every day."[98]

Plants Don't Contain Vitamin B12

The second argument often raised against switching to a plant-based diet concerns a vitamin that cannot be found in plant foods at all. There is no question that we need it. Dr. McDougall points out, "B12 is necessary for your nervous system and blood. Without adequate amounts of this vitamin in the body, anemia and degeneration of the nerves can occur."[99] Since vitamin B12 appears in some animal foods, the logic runs, we should be including plenty of animal foods in our diet.

To start, it should be pointed out that we don't need very much vitamin B12. Our body can store it for a long time, and we can go as long as three years without consuming any. Still, it seems strange that nature would not include a source for every essential nutrient in the natural diet for our species. Vitamin B12 is a specialized nutrient, not made by either animals or plants but by bacteria that live in the intestines of animals. Our prehistoric ancestors derived enough of these bacteria from the plants grown in soil containing the bacteria.

Nowadays, there are two obstacles to our getting enough B12. Many crops are grown in lifeless, overfertilized soil. In addition, modern hygiene practices remove all traces of dirt and bacteria on food before we eat it.

The solution to this problem is very simple for people who eat only whole plants. Many experts recommend an occasional B12 supplement. Dr. Barnard recommends another source, explaining that you will also find it in many "fortified products such as fortified breakfast cereals or fortified soy milk."[100] A quick check of the nutrition facts on the side of a cereal box will show you. To give you an idea how common this fortification practice is, a random check at the grocery store showed that four out of five cereals were fortified with vitamin B12.

Finally, Dr. Campbell weighs in with some straight talk from Chapter 11 of *The China Study*, "Though our society's obsession with nutrient supplements seriously detracts from other, far more important nutrition information, this is not to say that supplements should always be avoided. If you do not eat any animal products for three years or more, or are pregnant or breastfeeding, you should consider taking a small B12 supplement on occasion, or going to the doctor annually to check your blood levels of B vitamins."

We Need to Eat Fish for the Healthy Omega-3 Fatty Acids

Many would argue that eating fish is good for your heart and that fatty fish such as salmon is the best source of the heart-healthy omega-3 fatty acids. As Dr. Fuhrman says, "Optimal health depends on the proper balance of fatty acids in the diet . . . Our modern diet, full of vegetable oils and animal products, is very high in omega-6 fat and very low in omega-3 fat; the higher the omega-6 to omega-3 ratio, the higher the risk of heart disease, diabetes, and inflammatory illnesses."[101]

The question remains: is fish the best source for omega-3 fatty acids? Howard Lyman addresses this question in his book *No More Bull!* "Surely you've heard that fish, particularly fatty fish, is good for your heart. In fact, you've probably heard it about a million times."[102] But, he points out, there are other important facts to consider in this debate. "[E]ating fish will not prevent—indeed, it will assist—the slow, steady buildup of heart-destroying plaque in your arteries. Like meat, fish is a high-cholesterol 'food.' . . . Like meat, fish has no fiber. Like meat, fish offers no protective antioxidants, and little in the way of vitamins. Unfortunately, what fish does contain is enough mercury to help you take your temperature."[103]

Dr. Campbell also brings up a possible concern about consuming fish to get omega-3s. "If you've heard anything about omega-3 fatty acids, it's that you need more of them to be healthy," he says. Noting that you can't always believe what you hear on the evening news, he offers the following from a 1999 Harvard study: "[C]ontrary to the predominant hypothesis, we found an increased risk of breast cancer associated with omega-3 fats from fish."[104]

So where should we get the omega-3s that we need? It is a widely accepted fact that we do need to consume omega-3 fatty acids just like we must consume or manufacture all essential nutrients. But as with all other nutrients except vitamin B12, the best source is whole plants. In the case of omega-3s, two of the most convenient sources are ground flaxseed and walnuts. Most grocery stores sell either ground or whole flaxseed in bags. I keep my whole flaxseed in the refrigerator and use an old coffee grinder to prepare about a tablespoon for my cereal each morning. Table 3.2 provides an idea of how various plant-based sources stack up against fish.

Table 3.2 Foods Concentrated in Omega-3 Fatty Acids[105]

Food	Serving	Omega-3 Fatty Acids	Quality
Flaxseed	0.25 cup	7.0 g	Excellent
Walnuts	0.25 cup	2.3 g	Very good
Chinook salmon, baked/broiled	4.0 oz	2.1 g	Very good
Soybeans, cooked	1 cup	1.0 g	Good
Tofu, raw	4.0 oz	0.4 g	Good
Winter squash	1 cup	0.3 g	Good

We should also consider the fact that the benefit of omega-3s is not firmly established in scientific circles. While most experts would recommend their inclusion in the diet, Dr. Barnard cites scientific studies that challenge their overall effectiveness: "Omega-3 fats are reputed to reduce inflammation and block the formation of blood clots that could lead to heart attacks . . . Looking at 89 prior studies, the researchers found that whether omega-3 oils were consumed in fish or as supplements, they offered no significant protection against cardiovascular disease, cancer, or risk of death."[106]

We Need the Calcium in Dairy Products for Strong Bones

We touched on this topic in the previous chapter, but the information bears repeating here. For many people, calcium and strong bones are joined at the hip forever. The dairy industry has long promoted the consumption of milk so that we will get enough calcium to build strong bones and avoid osteoporosis. The argument is that if you don't drink milk, how could you possibly get enough calcium?

Sadly, numerous studies have shown that milk is actually one of the main causes of osteoporosis. Dr. Fuhrman points out one comparison: "American women drink thirty to thirty-two times as much cow's milk as the New Guineans, yet suffer forty-seven times as many broken hips."[107] Dr. McDougall cites another example:

> The African Bantu woman provides an excellent example of good health. Her diet is free of milk and still provides 250–400 mg of calcium per day from plant sources, which is one half the amount consumed by Western women. Bantu women commonly have ten babies during their life and breast feed each of them for about ten months. But even with this huge calcium drain and relatively low calcium intake, osteoporosis is relatively unknown among these women. It is interesting to note that when relatives of these same people migrate to the affluent societies and adopt rich diets, osteoporosis and diseases of the teeth become common.[108]

Dr. Campbell states in the movie *Forks over Knives*, "Cow's milk is nature's most perfect food—her most perfect food for baby cows, not for humans." After growing up on a dairy farm himself, he conducted scientific research on milk, cheese, and yogurt on a global basis. He points out that it just doesn't make any sense for us to be drinking cow's milk. We are the only species of animal that drinks the milk of another species. And we are the only species of animal that drinks any milk whatsoever after weaning.

This unnatural consumption of the animal protein (casein) in cow's milk may weaken bones and promote cancer. In *The China Study*, Dr. Campbell explains:

> We found that not all [animal] proteins had this [cancer-promoting] effect. What protein consistently and strongly promoted cancer? Casein, which makes up 87% of cow's milk protein, promoted all stages of the cancer process. What type of protein did not promote cancer, even at high levels of intake? The safe proteins were all from plants, including wheat and soy. As this picture came into view, it

began to challenge and then to shatter some of my most cherished assumptions.[109]

Is it hard to find calcium in other foods? Hardly. In fact, most brands of orange juice provide a calcium-fortified variety. Table 3.3 compares dairy and plant sources of calcium.

Table 3.3 Calcium in Dairy and Plant Foods[110]

Food	Calcium per Serving (mg)
Dairy products	
Skim milk (1 cup)	301
Whole milk (1 cup)	290
Plain low-fat yogurt (1 cup)	415
Cow milk cottage cheese (1 cup)	208
Buffalo milk cottage cheese (1 cup)	480
Beans and grains	
White beans (¾ cup)	120
Navy beans (¾ cup)	94
Black turtle beans (¾ cup)	75
Chickpeas (¾ cup)	58
Tofu (150 g)	350
Soy bean curd slab (150 g)	310
Cooked soybeans (1 cup)	130
Instant oats (1 packet)	165
Nuts	
Almonds, roasted (¼ cup)	93
Almond butter (2 tbsp)	88
Sesame seeds (¼ cup)	50
Vegetables and fruits	
Cabbage/bok choy (½ cup)	190
Turnip greens (½ cup)	104
Broccoli (½ cup)	33

Food	Calcium per Serving (mg)
Okra (½ cup)	65
Orange (½ cup)	52
Orange juice fortified with calcium (½ cup)	165

Milk Is the Best Source of Vitamin D

Many would argue that we need to drink milk to get enough vitamin D, which affects many parts of our body and its functions. What they don't realize is that very few foods in nature contain vitamin D—and milk is not one of them. Milk is artificially fortified with vitamin D during processing. The dairy industry made that decision long ago. The thinking was that, since everyone drinks milk, this is a surefire way to make sure everyone gets this critical vitamin, and it will help sell a lot more milk.

So where does vitamin D come from? Dr. Barnard clarifies the issue:

Technically, vitamin D is not a vitamin at all. It's actually a hormone produced by sunlight on your skin, which is then converted to its active forms as it passes through your liver and kidneys. Once activated, it helps you absorb calcium and helps protect your cells against cancer, among other functions. If you get plenty of sun, you do not need any vitamin D in your diet. Most of us are not that lucky, however. If you do not get regular sun exposure, taking a multivitamin containing 400 IU of vitamin D is important.[111]

Obtaining sufficient vitamin D from natural food sources alone can be difficult. For many people, consuming vitamin D–fortified foods and being exposed to sunlight are sufficient for maintaining a healthy level of vitamin D. In some groups, dietary supplements might be required to meet the daily need for vitamin D.

The Biggest Argument of All

As shown in the previous sections, the five nutritional arguments are easily answered with a simple review of the facts. The biggest argument of all against a plant-based diet, though, has nothing whatsoever to do with nutrition. It stems from the lack of recommendations from the medical community. Although many conventional medical doctors have become aware of the disease-reversal work by other doctors in the fields of heart disease and diabetes, among others, few have incorporated this new body of knowledge into their practice. Why not?

They have not been trained in what constitutes a health-promoting diet. In addition, most assume that the so-called optimal diet is too drastic for their patients and that their patients either would refuse to do it or would not be able to stick with it. In 1979, at the University of Kentucky, when Dr. James Anderson successfully reversed type 2 diabetes in many of his patients, he later commented that he felt that the diet required to achieve those results might be impractical for most patients. Medical doctors are not trained in nutrition and have not been coached on how to help patients overcome the psychological barriers associated with a dietary change that could possibly save their life. Doctors may have confidence in the health-promoting power of a whole-foods, plant-based diet, but they are not comfortable or knowledgeable enough to influence their patients. Dr. McDougall explains:

> As a rule, doctors do not dispense good nutrition information. Part of the reason may be that only a minority of physicians receive any training in nutrition while they are in medical school. Currently, only 29 of the 129 medical schools in the United States have required nutrition education courses. A 1993 survey of 30,000 physician-members of the American Medical Association (with 3,400 responding) found that less than one-quarter of doctors actually ask their patients about their diets, and only one-third of them incorporate nutritional information in their practice.[112]

An eighty-five-year-old friend of mine told me recently that not a single doctor had ever asked him about his diet.

Dr. Esselstyn would argue that doctors everywhere should explain as best they can all of the options open to any individual patient and then let their patients decide if a diet is too drastic. As he said in a recent lecture at our club, "Certainly many patients might consider eating broccoli and Brussels sprouts not nearly as severe as opening up their chest for bypass surgery." To be fair, the medical doctors within the system are not to be blamed; they likely went to medical school for the right reasons and are simply doing their best to help people by performing the diagnoses, writing the prescriptions, and conducting the procedures that they have been taught.

Finally, there is one other category of resistance that you will likely encounter when moving from the typical Western diet to a health-promoting, plant-based diet. We refer to the obstacles of this category as "social barriers" and will address them in Chapter 10.

> "People often say that humans have always eaten animals, as if this is some justification for continuing the practice. According to this logic, we should not try to prevent people from murdering other people, since this has also been done since the earliest of times."
>
> —Isaac Bashevis Singer

PART II

What You Eat Affects Far More Than Just Your Health

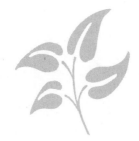

4

RUNNING ROUGHSHOD

"The nation that destroys its soil destroys itself."

—Franklin D. Roosevelt

During my high school years in semirural Tennessee, I had the opportunity to experience firsthand raising livestock. My father oversaw several farms in the area, including one dairy farm and another that raised broiler chickens, and I spent a lot of time on each.

When it was my day to handle the early-morning milking of our herd of thirty-five Holsteins, I would rise at 4:00 AM before going to school, drive out to the farm, and begin herding all the cows into the holding area next to the milking barn. While congregated in this area and at times while in the milking barn, the cows would relieve themselves as they pleased. This fresh manure would be hand-shoveled into a spreader parked next to the holding area. Every few weeks, whenever the spreader was filled to overflowing, we would use the tractor to haul it through either the pasture or croplands right there on the farm, enriching the soil in the age-old farmer's cycle.

A similar process took place at the chicken farm. After the growth period for the 5,000 birds ended and they were shipped off to market, we would haul a manure spreader into the barn, where we would scoop up the dried manure that was piled about six inches high throughout the barn. With two of us shoveling, filling the spreader would take about thirty minutes, and then it would be hauled by tractor through the fields.

Looking back, I would call both farms a model of "green" livestock farming. The entire process served to protect the soil, the water supply, and our climate. Our little farms were among thousands of similar farms around the country at that time. The situation has changed dramatically since those days. For the most part, small family farms have been replaced by mega factory farms. These agribusiness holdings have steadily taken over growing the animals required as the world has increasingly adopted the typical meat-heavy Western diet. According to the USDA, in the United States alone, yearly chicken consumption per person has risen from ten pounds in the late 1940s to almost sixty pounds in 2000—a 600 percent increase in just fifty years.[113]

These changes are happening on a global basis as well. The *New York Times* reported in 2008:

> Global demand for meat has multiplied in recent years, encouraged by growing affluence and nourished by the proliferation of huge, confined animal feeding operations. These assembly-line meat factories consume enormous amounts of energy, pollute water supplies, generate significant greenhouse gases and require ever-increasing amounts of corn, soy and other grains, a dependency that has led to the destruction of vast swaths of the world's tropical rain forests.[114]

The article goes on to report that the world's total meat production had risen 400 percent since 1961—from 71 million tons to 284 million tons in 2007. Personal consumption doubled during that period and is expected to double again by 2050.

Currently, the United States grows and kills about 10 billion animals per year, a little over 15 percent of the global total of 60 billion, a number that is expected to double to 120 billion by 2050.[115] Where does the proliferation end? As Jonathan Foer points out in his book *Eating Animals*, "If the world followed America's lead, we would consume over 165 billion chickens annually (even if the population didn't increase)."[116]

A handful of those little farms of my youth still exist, but they are declining in number every year. The domination of agribusiness giants extends across the spectrum of animals grown for human consumption, including cattle. Eric Schlosser in *Fast Food Nation* remarks on the gap between pioneer lore and reality:

> Ranchers and cowboys have long been the central icons of the American West. Traditionalists have revered them as symbols of freedom and self-reliance . . . [Yet] American ranchers . . . are rapidly disappearing. Over the last twenty years, about half a million ranchers sold off their cattle and quit the business. Many of the nation's remaining eight hundred thousand ranchers are faring poorly . . . The sort of hard-working ranchers long idealized in cowboy myths are the ones most likely to go broke today.[117]

Anna Lappé in *Diet for a Hot Planet* relates how only a handful of giants have come to control vast proportions of food-animal production: "By 2007, Tyson, Cargill, Swift & Co. (now owned by Brazilian company, JBS) and National Packing Co. controlled 84.5 percent of beef packing operations. In the business of broilers (non–egg laying poultry), Pilgrim's Pride, Tyson, Perdue, and Sanderson Farms controlled 58.5 percent of the market."[118] While factory farms have been very good for the pocketbook of consumers, they have not been so kind to the health of those consumers—or to the health of the global environment.

What Is a Factory Farm?

Actually, agribusinesses hate the term "factory farm," because it too accurately describes how their animals are treated. The official name is a CAFO (pronounced KAY-foe)—a contained animal feeding operation. CAFOs account for the vast majority of the production of beef, pork, eggs, milk, turkey, and chicken—and most of them are owned by huge corporations. To be able to compete at the supermarket register, these farms must simply be too large to be managed by a single family. Since the vast majority of our meat, dairy, and egg appetites are being fed by these types of farms, with few exceptions, the small family-managed farm that I remember has gone the way of the manual typewriter.

As Jonathan Foer reports, "For each food animal species, animal agriculture is now dominated by the factory farm—99.9 percent of the chickens raised for meat, 96 percent of laying hens, 99 percent of turkeys, 95 percent of pigs, and 78 percent of cattle."[119] You do have the choice of buying free-range chickens or grass-fed beef, but they're both essentially novelty items today. Thanks to the highly engineered factory farm, the people of the Western world are now able to afford animal-based foods three meals a day.

So what happened to those millions of bucolic farms of yore? They were the victim of two developments: a free market system and a never-ending process of continuous improvement—delivering more product for less money. The free market system will always work to deliver what consumers want, and companies compete for market share by becoming more efficient. The capitalist system works very well in most product categories but not so well in the world of the factory farm. That's because the unit of production is a living, breathing animal or the eggs or milk that are taken from an animal. In their continual quest for lower prices and more profits, factory farms have "engineered" every element of the process—beginning with genetically designing the perfect broiler, the perfect laying hen, the perfect pig, or the perfect cow. Perfect in this case doesn't mean healthy; it just means that it has the desired taste, it grows fast, and it is produced with ever increasing efficiency. The producers hope that these "perfect" animals will stay alive long enough to be slaughtered and sold as food for people. But because of the many hazards of their short, unhealthy lives, many of them die in the process. Those unfortunates become a part of the reusable waste that will eventually be fed to other farm animals.

The problems associated with mass-producing these "perfect" animals are widespread. To maximize production, each farm raises thousands of animals in very small spaces where many of them never see the light of day. They are given growth hormones and antibiotics to make them grow quickly and keep them alive within these cramped environments that are prone to contagion. The amount of excrement that these animals produce is a monumental environmental concern. As Foer reports, "Today a typical pig factory farm will produce 7.2 million pounds of manure annually, a typical broiler facility will produce 6.6 million pounds, and a typical cattle feedlot 344 million pounds. All told, farmed animals in the United States produce 130 times as much waste as the human population—roughly 87,000 pounds of [solid waste] *per second*."[120] These numbers are very difficult to fully comprehend, so let's think of them in another way. If we do a little math, that converts to a staggering 1.37 billion tons of animal waste each year. That works out to almost 9,000 pounds for every human being in the United States. Want a visualization of that amount? How would you like to see your share pull into your driveway? That would be nine pickup trucks filled to overflowing. Got a family of four? You better have a big driveway, because you're going to need thirty-six trucks to hold your family's share of this mess. And this incredible environmental problem is getting worse all the time.

So what else goes on at the typical factory farm? Well, that's some dirt the entire industry would like to keep secret, and we'll talk more about the treatment of the animals in Chapter 7. But from an environmental standpoint, the factory farm's efficiency is anything but a bargain. It causes alarming degradation of the world's arable land (land that can be used for growing crops), recklessly uses and pollutes our water supply, and negatively affects the climate and biodiversity. The factory farm does indeed produce cheap food—that is, until you factor in the damage to our environment.

Livestock's impact on the world's environmental health became the focus of a major study by the United Nations, which released its findings in a report titled *Livestock's Long Shadow* in November 2006. The report advocates a major policy focus on a host of problems. "Livestock's contribution to environmental problems is on a massive scale and its potential contribution to their solution is equally large. The impact is so significant that it needs to be addressed with urgency."[121] The report focuses on four categories of environmental damage that stems from the raising of livestock for our dinner tables: land degradation and deforestation, atmosphere and climate, water shortage and pollution, and biodiversity and the loss of species.

Land Degradation and Deforestation

Land is critical in any conversation about the environment. After all, whether we are eating sirloin or spinach, we need land to produce our food. The problem is that we need a lot more of it to produce the sirloin. Whether we are burning precious rain forests in Brazil to make room for grazing cattle or destroying our topsoil to create feed for beef, we're devastating land at record speed, and this is clearly a serious problem. The following are some major points of the UN report.

- In all, raising livestock accounts for 78 percent of all agricultural land and 30 percent of the land surface of the planet.[122]
- Expansion of livestock production is a key factor in deforestation, especially in Latin America, where the greatest amount of

deforestation is occurring. Seventy percent of previously for-
ested land in the Amazon is occupied by pastures, and feed
crops cover a large part of the remainder. [123]

- About 20 percent of the world's pastures and rangelands, with
  73 percent of rangelands in dry areas, have been degraded to
  some extent, mostly through overgrazing, compaction, and
  erosion created by livestock.[124]

We have been hearing about these problems for over thirty years, but
the situation continues to worsen—all over the world. Back in 1987,
John Robbins reported a host of facts on this topic in *Diet for a New
America*. Back then, the U.S. Soil Conservation Service reported that
over 4 million acres (an area about the size of Connecticut) of cropland
were being lost to erosion in this country each year, equating to an
annual topsoil loss of 7 billion tons. Of this staggering loss, 85 percent
was associated with the raising of livestock.[125] How so? According to
a 2010 University of Michigan Global Change Program document, the
top three causes of soil degradation are overgrazing, agricultural activities (lack of sustainable organic practices), and deforestation.[126] The
lion's share is related to the world's appetite for meat.

Dr. David Pimentel of Cornell University comments on the severity
of the problem as well:

> The United States is losing soil 10 times faster—and China and India
> are losing soil 30 to 40 times faster—than the natural replenishment
> rate. As a result of erosion over the past 40 years, 30 percent of
> the world's arable land has become unproductive. About 60 percent
> of soil that is washed away ends up in rivers, streams and lakes,
> making waterways more prone to flooding and to contamination
> from soil's fertilizers and pesticides.[127]

It would be nice if the problem were confined to the poor beasts
raised on factory farms. Grass-fed cattle roam free, right? Yes, and

while they enjoy a much better life than the CAFO animal, their grazing is still environmentally destructive. Although we don't have to
devote vast amounts of land to raising their food, grass-fed cattle have
been taking their toll on the Earth's surface for over two millennia. In
his 1998 book, former cattle rancher Howard F. Lyman sums up the
global overgrazing situation: "By introducing cattle in unnatural numbers onto marginal land where they do not belong in the first place, we
are tampering dangerously with complex ecosystems."[128]

Lyman further points out that the Earth's surface was not originally
designed for cattle grazing, and the land out West that is marginal for
growing crops has been deteriorating ever since the first cowboys:

> [M]ore than half of western topsoil has been lost since livestock
> began overtaking the western plains 140 years ago. Topsoil is the
> most precious commodity a farmer has. It takes Nature anywhere
> between one hundred and eight hundred years to produce one inch
> of topsoil. Since the founding of the United States, Nature would
> have provided us with, at most, about two inches more of topsoil,
> but due to our chemical farming practices and our essential for-
> feiture of sovereignty over the land to cattle, we've lost about six
> inches. We are squandering a resource whose preciousness we don't
> even begin to understand, and floods are just part of our collective
> comeuppance.[129]

As noted previously, the problem isn't confined to the United States.
The greatest destruction by far has occurred in Brazil, where a price-
less resource is being lost. According to estimates, roughly a fifth of
the Amazon rain forest, an area the size of California, has been lost
since the 1970s. That has helped make Brazil's agribusiness corpora-
tion JBS become the largest meat supplier in the world.

What can be done to slow down or stop this environmental devasta-
tion? Cornell researchers estimate that for every person who eliminates
animal foods from his or her diet, an acre of trees is spared every year.[130]

Right now, there are roughly 10 million Americans (3.2 percent) who consider themselves vegetarian. With growing awareness, that number could easily double or triple in the next few years. When 20 million more Americans switch to a primarily plant-based diet, it will save close to 20 million acres of trees, an area about the size of Indiana.

Atmosphere and Climate

In the summer of 2006, just before the release of the UN report previously mentioned, former vice president Al Gore starred in the movie *An Inconvenient Truth*, which sounded a clarion call about the looming disaster the world may face if it cannot halt human-made global warming. Though the movie was effective in sounding the alarm, it is curious that Gore failed to mention that the raising of livestock is one of the leading causes of greenhouse gases—having a larger impact than *all* transportation combined. That's right; the livestock sector accounts for roughly a third more gases than all those highway exhaust fumes.

As it relates to atmosphere and climate, the UN report points out several problems with raising livestock. The livestock sector is responsible for 18 percent of all greenhouse gas emissions, measured in carbon dioxide equivalents, which includes not only CO_2 but also methane and nitrous oxide. In contrast, transportation (mainly automobiles) accounts for only 13.5 percent of the total. Livestock create 9 percent of the CO_2; 37 percent of all methane, a deadly gas with 23 times the global warming potential of CO_2; and 65 percent of all nitrous oxide, which has a global warming potential 296 times that of CO_2 and also contributes to acid rain.[131] Most of this nitrous oxide comes from manure. A recent study published in *Science* magazine found that this gas is the single most important ozone-depleting substance (ODS) and is expected to remain the most abundant throughout the twenty-first century.[132] Livestock are also responsible for almost two-thirds of anthropogenic (human-caused) methane emissions, mainly through belching and releases of intestinal gas, which contribute significantly to acid rain and acidification of ecosystems. According to Howard Lyman, every cow emits up to 400 quarts of methane gas per day.[133]

In addition to these greenhouse gases, the livestock sector leads all human-produced sources in ammonia emissions (accounting for 64 percent of the world's total). Ammonia also contributes significantly to acid rain and acidification of ecosystems. According to the UN report, the largest source of atmospheric ammonia is from the decay of organic matter in soils—an estimated 50 million tons per year. An estimated 23 million of those tons are produced by domesticated animals. This compares to only 3 million tons from all the wild animals of the world.[134]

Beyond all the big numbers, the crisis boils down to a single problem. Too many animals are populating the world, an offshoot of the problem of human overpopulation. But while the upward curve of the human population is expected to level off, the curve of animals raised for food is poised to shoot exponentially higher. We could all switch to electric vehicles—every one of us—and still the world would grow hotter because of those bites at the end of our forks.

Water Shortage and Pollution

Our water supply is one of the favorite topics of environmentalists around the world—and it should be. The UN report projects that 64 percent of the world's population will live in water-stressed basins by 2025. According to a 2008 UNEP Report, "Agricultural water use accounts for about 75% of total global consumption (mainly for crop irrigation), while industrial use accounts for about 20%, and the remaining 5% is used for domestic purposes."[135] Some striking numbers from *When the Rivers Run Dry*: "It takes 3,000 gallons to grow the feed for enough cow to make a quarter-pound hamburger, and between

500 and 1,000 gallons for that cow to fill its udders with a quart of milk. Cheese? That takes about 650 gallons for a pound of cheddar or brie or camembert."[136]

An estimated 70 percent of all of the water used in the eleven western states of the United States is dedicated to the raising of animals for food. Much of that water comes from the largest underground lake in the world, the Ogallala Aquifer, which reaches from Texas to South Dakota and from Missouri to Colorado. About half the grain-fed cattle in America depend on water from this great aquifer to irrigate their feed crops, which contributes mightily to the three cubic miles of water that have been drained annually from this reserve for the past forty years. It took millions of years to create the lake, but at the current rate of consumption, this great natural resource will be mostly exhausted by 2050.[137]

The depletion of underground aquifers is a rapidly growing problem across the globe. Fred Pearce visited a small dairy farmer in India, where wells are increasingly coming up dry. Pearce says, "He has a small pump that brings to the surface 3,200 gallons of water an hour . . . mostly to grow alfalfa to feed his cows. His farm's main output is 6.5 gallons of milk a day. I did the math. He uses 4.8 million gallons of water a year to grow the fodder to produce just over 2,400 gallons of milk. That's 2,000 gallons of water for every gallon of milk."[138] This same inefficiency is replicated at countless dairies worldwide, and the problem is the same. Water that is pumped out of the ground will run out someday—and in most places in the world, sooner rather than later.

Water.org reports that nearly 1 billion people lack access to safe water, and 2.5 billion do not have improved sanitation. The health and economic impacts are staggering. More people in the world own cell phones than have access to a toilet. And as cities and slums grow at increasing rates, the situation worsens. Every day, lack of access to clean water and sanitation kills thousands and leaves others with a poor quality of life.

How can we save our water? Soil and water specialists at the University of California Agricultural Extension in 1978 found that to produce one pound of California beef, it takes 5,214 gallons of water[139]—the amount of water required for one full year of seven-minute showers. Howard Lyman makes a telling point in *Mad Cowboy*:

> We often hear about water shortages in areas such as Southern California, where citizens are recurrently requested not to wash their cars, not to overwater their lawns, and to use the low-flow showers and toilets. Good ideas, all. But you never hear city, county, or state governments combating drought by urging their citizens to cut down on meat consumption, even though the water required to produce *just ten pounds of steak* equals the water consumption of the average household for a year.[140]

John Robbins offers a simple solution in line with Lyman's ideas: "You see people who are environmentalists trying to conserve water washing their cars less often, installing low flow sinks and toilets, drought resistant landscaping, and legislation passing requiring low flow shower heads and so forth. These are all prudent and helpful measures, but all combined they don't even compare to what you save by eating one less hamburger."[141]

In the great 2009 movie *HOME*, produced in France by PPR, Glenn Close told us some pretty scary numbers relative to the water use efficiency of producing meat. "To produce one kilo of potatoes requires 100 litres of water; to produce the same amount of beef requires 13,000 litres of water. Converting those numbers to water comsumption per calorie, we find that it takes over 75 times as much water to produce a calorie of beef compared to the potato. John Robbins provides similar data in *The Food Revolution* for a wide array of fruits, vegetables, and meats. From those numbers, we determined that while beef is the least efficient of the meats; on average it takes more than twenty times more water (per calorie) to produce meat compared to whole, plant-based foods.

Not only are livestock using huge quantities of water; they're also polluting it. On the traditional farm, a cow patty represents a means of returning nutrients to the soil. But the numbers of animals confined on factory farms defecate in quantities that far surpass the farm's ability to dispose of them. This problem has led some farms to use wholly inadequate systems of removal, which have led to environmental disasters all across the country.

In *Eating Animals*, Jonathan Foer summarizes the crux of the problem. The U.S. General Accounting Office (GAO) reports that individual CAFOs can generate more waste than the populations of some U.S. cities. Amazingly, the polluting strength of the CAFO waste is 160 times greater than that of raw municipal sewage. "And yet there is almost no waste-treatment infrastructure for farmed animals—no toilets, obviously, but also no sewage pipes, no one hauling it away for treatment, and almost no federal guidelines regulating what happens to it."[142]

The implications for human health are obvious. As David Kirby relates in *Animal Factory*, "While human sewage is treated to kill pathogens, animal waste is not. Hog manure has ten to one hundred times more concentrated pathogens than human waste, yet the law would never permit untreated human waste to be kept in vast 'lagoons,' or sprayed onto fields, as is the case with manure."[143]

Remember that 1.37 billion tons of animal excrement produced annually in just the United States? What happens to this massive amount of dangerous animal waste? The short answer is that it ends up in our water supply. The EPA estimates that chicken, hog, and cattle excrement has already polluted thousands of miles of rivers. These assaults on the water supply have not gone unnoticed. In 1995, a malfunctioning manure lagoon at SNB Farms in Webster City, Iowa, spilled 1.5 million gallons of manure into the South Fork of the Iowa River. Within one week in 1998, two dairies in Washington State had separate spills that dumped 2 million gallons of manure into the Yakima River. In 2005, Oklahoma's attorney general sued thirteen poultry companies, claiming they had damaged one of the state's most important watersheds. A report of the Natural Resources Defense Council cites multiple abuses in thirty states.[144] The list goes on and on.

The largest spill occurred in North Carolina, a state that since the 1990s has been overrun by industrial hog farms, dominated by Smithfield, the largest hog agribusiness in the country. In his *Rolling Stone* article "Boss Hog" Jeff Tietz describes the terrible disaster:

> The biggest spill in the history of corporate hog farming happened in 1995. The dike of a 120,000-square-foot lagoon owned by a Smithfield competitor ruptured, releasing 25.8 million gallons of effluvium into the headwaters of the New River in North Carolina. It was the biggest environmental spill in United States history, more than twice as big as the Exxon Valdez oil spill six years earlier. The sludge was so toxic it burned your skin if you touched it, and so dense it took almost two months to make its way sixteen miles downstream to the ocean. From the headwaters to the sea, every creature living in the river was killed. Fish died by the millions.[145]

A September 2009 article in the *New York Times* reports, "Agricultural runoff is the single largest source of water pollution in the nation's rivers and streams, according to the E.P.A. An estimated 19.5 million Americans fall ill each year from waterborne parasites, viruses or bacteria, including those stemming from human and animal waste."[146]

Sometimes large figures like these are hard to wrap our mind around. Let's look at a fairly run-of-the-mill spill in Morrison, Wisconsin, a state famous for its dairy farms. In the same *Times* article, one neighbor told what happened to her. "[M]ore than 100 wells were polluted by agricultural runoff within a few months, according to local officials. As parasites and bacteria seeped into drinking water, residents suffered from chronic diarrhea, stomach illnesses and severe ear infections. 'Sometimes it smells like a barn coming out of the faucet,' said Lisa Barnard, who lives a few towns over."[147]

Although millions of farmers have been displaced by the growth of CAFOs during the last fifty years, some of them are still running smaller niche market farms that specialize in the ethical treatment of animals. Jonathan Foer tells the story of one such pork farmer and how he and his wife had planned to retire at a small farm nearby one day. After years of preparing their "dream farm" for that retirement, they learned that a CAFO hog farm (holding 6,000 hogs) would soon be built on the land adjacent to their planned home.

Next to their dream, now, loomed a nightmare: thousands of suffering, sick hogs surrounded by, and themselves suffering within, a thick, nausea-inducing stench. Not only will the nearby factory farm decimate Paul's land's value (estimates suggest land degradation from industrial farming has cost Americans $26 billion) and destroy the land itself, not only will the smell make cohabitation incredibly unpleasant at best and more likely dangerous to Paul's family's health, but it stands in opposition to everything Paul has spent his life working for.[148]

The United States is not the only place where agricultural abuses occur. Smithfield, the hog king, has moved into eastern Europe in a big way. A May 2009 *New York Times* article explains the effect: "With almost 40 farms in western Romania, Smithfield has built enormous metal manure containers to inject waste into the soil. 'We go crazy with the daily smell,' said Aura Danielescu, the principal of a school in Masloc, who closes her windows tight. Smithfield farms in Romania's Timis County are among the top sources of air and soil pollution, according to a local government report, which ranked the company's individual farms No. 13 through No. 40. The report also indicates that methane gases in the air rose 65 percent between 2002 and 2007."[149]

Disturbing reports like these continue to mount. What will it take for governments to step in and impose regulations to safeguard our health? What will it take for people to demand safety over cheap bacon? The probable truth is that only a disaster that kills humans rather than fish will wake us up to the industrial-food time bombs tucked away in our pastoral countryside.

Biodiversity and the Loss of Species

Why is biodiversity so important? An environment's biodiversity is determined by the number of different animal and plant species that live in it. Rich biodiversity is crucial to the structure of the ecosystems and habitats that support all living things—including wildlife, fish, and forests. The greater the number of different species of plants and animals, the healthier the ecosystem and the better able to withstand disaster it is. Biodiversity helps provide for our basic human needs such as food, shelter, and medicine, all of which are derived (directly or indirectly) from biological sources, and it fosters ecosystems that maintain oxygen in the air, enrich the soil, and purify the water. Strong ecosystems help to protect against flood and storm damage and regulate climate. In a nutshell, biodiversity makes sustained living on planet Earth possible for all living creatures.

What is happening to our biodiversity and why? Our rapid consumption of resources and growing populations have led to a loss of other forms of life, which has disrupted ecosystems across the world. This loss has eroded the capacity of Earth's natural systems to provide essential elements that humans depend on. Human activities have raised the rate of extinction to 1,000 times its usual rate. If we continue on this path, Earth will experience the sixth great wave of extinctions in billions of years of history.[150]

We're seeing dramatic evidence of problems that the human race has created in the past century. According to the previously mentioned UN report, we are in an era of unprecedented threats to biodiversity. The rate at which we're losing species is estimated to be fifty to five hundred times higher than historical rates found in the fossil record. Fifteen out of twenty-four important ecosystem services are assessed to be in decline. *The livestock sector may well be the leading player in the reduction of biodiversity*, since it is a major driver of deforestation, land degradation, pollution, climate change, overfishing, sedimentation of coastal areas, and facilitation of invasions by alien species.[151] Conservation International has identified thirty-five global hot spots for biodiversity, characterized by exceptional levels of plant endemism and serious levels of habitat loss. Of these, twenty-three are reported to be affected by livestock production. An analysis of the authoritative International Union for Conservation of Nature (IUCN) Red List of Threatened Species shows that most of the world's threatened species are suffering habitat loss where livestock are a factor.[152]

An estimated two of every three bird species in the world are in decline; one in every eight plant species is endangered or threatened; and one-quarter of mammals, one-quarter of amphibians, and one-fifth of reptiles are endangered or vulnerable.[153] Also in crisis are forests and fisheries, which are essential biological resources and integral parts of the Earth's ecosystems. Forests are home to 50 to 90 percent of terrestrial species. They also provide services such as carbon storage and flood prevention, and they are critical resources for many culturally diverse societies and millions of indigenous people. The World Resources Institute estimates that only one-fifth of the Earth's original forest cover has survived, and still deforestation continues, with 445 million acres in developing countries deforested between 1980 and 1995.[154]

John Robbins comments on the extent of this loss of habitat: "[The n]umber of species of birds in one square mile of Amazon rainforest [is] more than exists in all of North America . . . The number one factor in elimination of Latin America's tropical rain forests is cattle grazing . . . Every second, an area the size of a football field is destroyed forever."[155] How much species extinction is normal? Biologists esti-mate that the normal rate of extinctions is about ten to twenty-five species per year. We are, however, now losing at least several thousand species a year, and possibly tens of thousands.[156]

Our forests aren't the only habitats in trouble; marine ecosystems are in danger as well. Overfishing, destructive fishing techniques, and other human activities have severely jeopardized the health of many of the world's fish stocks along with associated marine species and eco-systems. The UN Food and Agriculture Organization estimates that more than half of ocean fish stocks are exploited at or beyond capac-ity.[157] At the same time, our agricultural practices on land are begin-ning to foul the oceans as well.

Dr. Bruce Monger, who teaches oceanography at Cornell Univer-sity, has uncovered some alarming facts on this pollution. After plot-ting the explosive growth of human population, the increase of CO_2 in the atmosphere, the escalation of deforestation, and the increase in the use of industrial nitrogen fertilizer from 1980 to 2009—all on the same graph—he was "blown away" by what he saw. In a 2009 online lecture, he exclaimed, "Boy, I've got to get interested in what's going on with nitrogen, because it's by far the most rapidly increasing item of this group."[158] Some estimate that we've put more nitrogen-based fertilizer in the ground in the last twenty years than we've put in the ground since fertilizer was invented. This unprecedented increase in the use of chemical fertilizer has been driven in large part by the crops grown to feed the billions of CAFO animals. Just as their manure pollutes our rivers and streams, the fertilizer used to grow their feed is beginning to do a number on our oceans. As Dr. Monger explains:

> When you have heavy agriculture and you pour large amounts of fertilizer on the land . . . a large fraction washes off the land into streams and is eventually brought to the coastal ocean, where it's dumped . . . That nitrogen in turn stimulates exceptionally strong growth by algae, which creates an exceptionally large biomass of

algae in the surface water. This algae eventually dies and usually sinks into coastal waters, typically near river outflows. Bacteria consume that dead algae for food, and they consume the oxygen in the water along with it. The more nutrients you dump in the ocean from land, the more algae, and the more bacteria consume oxygen until the oxygen in the water falls to near zero.[159]

After a few more steps, this process leads to what oceanographers call dead zones, areas of very low or zero oxygen where nothing that uses oxygen for growth can live. Dr. Monger goes on to explain that this is a problem not only for the Mississippi River or for the United States but for the entire world. The same blights we see along the Gulf and East Coast of the United States we see in Europe, South America, Asia, and Australia.

Fish farming is another industry that has enjoyed unprecedented growth in recent years, which contributes to the problem globally. As we discuss in Chapter 7, these floating CAFOs are no picnic for the poor fish, and they're equally bad for the environment—primarily because of the nitrogen used for these farms. As Dr. Monger says, "Farmed fish need to be fed something. If you're growing salmon in a pen off the coast, you have to dump fish food in there, and that fish food is full of nitrogen, and a lot of the food won't be consumed, and the fish will excrete it."[160] So the problem of nitrogen pollution is compounded, and unlike the nitrogen from fertilizer, the nitrogen from the fish farms doesn't have to travel down streams and rivers first. It bleeds directly into the ocean.

Everything Is Connected

When humankind discovered centuries ago that we live on a spherical planet, we started down the road of becoming aware that the Earth is a whole system in which all parts are connected. The plethora of global environmental issues we are experiencing today is constantly driving home that point. To summarize our dilemma, the world already has too many people, yet we continue to grow at a rapid rate. On top of that, the developing world is rapidly adopting the highly inefficient and environmentally destructive Western diet. The land available to feed the world is decreasing every year, which drives us to continue to *run roughshod* over the planet in the search of more land. With the desertification of former farmlands continuing at a frightening rate around the world, the prognosis for our sustained ability to feed the world is downright scary (we discuss this further in Chapter 6). And let's not forget the problems associated with our water supply, the loss of species, and the looming issue of global warming.

The sum total of our dilemma is mind-boggling. But a large part of the solution is refreshingly simple. John Robbins sums it up well:

> We undermine our own survival if we pollute our air and water, if we destroy the rainforests and deplete our natural resources . . . Increasing numbers of people today are aware of the need to honor the Earth and . . . to reduce . . . our "ecological footprint." . . . [Yet f]ew of us realize there is something we all could do that would have a tremendous impact on reducing pollution, conserving resources, and protecting our precious planet and the life it holds. There is indeed one action, within the grasp of each and every one of us, that could help to turn the tide. And yet most of us don't know what it is. I am talking about what you eat.[161]

Collectively, we have created a global crisis in the past century, and collectively, we need to fix it. For that we need leadership, but unfortunately, most of our leaders, even those few who might understand the devastating environmental impact of our Western diet, have apparently concluded that a planned, deliberate move away from it is unrealistic. I hear it all the time. Lots of people have heard that eating meat causes much of global warming and other environmental problems, but they think it would be too extreme, too radical or unrealistic, to try to adopt a plant-based diet.

Fortunately, that feeling is beginning to change, and the grassroots movement that is driving the change received a shot in the arm in September 2010 when Bill Clinton announced that he had starting eating a plant-based diet. Although he didn't do it for environmental reasons, the fact that he switched over will convince millions of people worldwide that his new diet could possibly be realistic after all. With a few more high-profile endorsements like this one, the widespread return to the natural diet for our species will gather momentum.

Approximately 1 million additional Americans are shifting to a primarily plant-based diet each year. Many of them are college students, who are six times more likely to be vegetarian than all other adults in the country. As we know, college students love to get behind what they consider positive change. Just as they helped to elect Barack Obama president, these educated young people will be major players in this critical process of inevitable change. Humans must ultimately become more environmentally responsible citizens of the world. We have already reached the breaking point for the cost of health-care in much of the world; likewise, we'll soon reach a breaking point for many environmental issues. To continue down our current path is simply no longer an option. It is overwhelmingly unsustainable.

"We do not inherit the land from our ancestors; we borrow it from our children."

—Native American proverb

5

THE END OF CHEAP OIL

"The frog does not drink up the pond in which he lives."

—Buddhist proverb

Disaster and tragedy are two words that come to mind when you think of the 2010 BP oil spill in the Gulf of Mexico. The spill and the associated threat to the nearby coastlines captured news headlines for months, prompting some analysts to worry that this massive spill might send the price of oil through the roof. Why did that not happen? It turns out that even though the spill caused a tremendous amount of environmental and economic damage, the quantity of oil lost was only a drop in the bucket of the world's daily consumption.

A few months after the blowout occurred, the U.S. government estimated that the total amount of oil that had spilled was between 88 million and 174 million gallons.[162] Even the high end of that range equals just over 4 million barrels of oil (at forty-two gallons per barrel)—a sizeable amount for sure but less than 5 percent of the world's daily consumption of oil. That means that after eighty-seven days of nonstop oil spewing, the total amount lost was enough to satisfy only a single hour of the world's thirst for this finite natural resource—a hefty 3.7 billion gallons per day (almost 90 million barrels).[163]

The BP spill is significant for two reasons. First, the fact that an oil company would dig a well a mile into the ocean floor shows how hard oil companies all over the world are trying to maintain the supply of oil. The supply side of the oil equation worries many experts, who point out that the known reserves are declining and will not last forever. But its continued flow for the next thirty or forty years is crucial. With more people on the planet and more of them driving cars, it's unlikely that we'll be able to significantly reduce usage for transportation and home heating. Second, the spill illustrates just how wasteful we are about using oil.

As Jeff Rubin, author of *Why Your World Is about to Get a Whole Lot Smaller*, points out, even with all the energy-saving devices being introduced, the numbers for fossil fuel consumption keep getting worse. "Despite the fact that the world is quickly waking up to the problem, emissions in the first decade of the millennium are growing four times faster than they did in the 1990s."[164] We understand the problem, but we aren't aware of all of the possible solutions.

What does oil have to do with food? While everybody knows that oil consumption could be reduced by driving a fuel-efficient car, very few realize how much energy is required to produce food these days. By simply altering our choices of what we eat, we could make significant savings in oil consumption. Once again, as we found with water in the last chapter, our plant-based calories are far more efficient to produce compared to the calories that are derived from meat and dairy. The production of animal foods for our dinner table is one of the single largest consumers of energy. Jeff Rubin observes, "We may think of farms as rustic Edens of placid cows in bucolic pastures and merry chickens pecking away in the barnyard, but behind that green facade is one of the most energy-intensive industries in the world. Large-scale, mechanized commercial farming is just a sophisticated way of turning fossil fuels into food."[165]

Julian Cribb, author of *The Coming Famine*, makes a similar point: "Most people haven't a clue how much oil they eat. For a person on a typical Western diet, one estimate is around 4.4 liters (about 1.2 U.S. gallons) of diesel a day, meaning that it takes the distillate from 66 barrels of crude oil just to put their food on the table for a year. A well-off family consisting of two parents and two children 'eats' 175 barrels of oil—almost one barrel every two days."[166]

The idea of eating oil is not a particularly pleasant one, but the point is that oil is vital to modern farming practices. That tractors need fuel is obvious, but other needs are not so apparent. Bill McKibben, a prominent writer on the environment, points them out in his book *Deep Economy*. "It takes half a gallon of oil to produce a bushel of midwestern hybrid corn; a quarter of it is used to make fertilizer, 35 percent to power the farm machinery, 7 percent to irrigate the field, and the rest to make pesticides, to dry grain, and to perform all the other tasks of industrial farming." That's only to grow the crop, however. He goes on: "But farming proper is the least of it. Processing, packaging, and distributing the food around the nation and the world consume four times again as much energy."[167]

Unless you shop at your local farmers' market, most of the meat you buy—wrapped in plastic and stacked in white bins at the supermarket—is part of a well-oiled system. We demand this vast supermarket selection because we have become accustomed to endless variety for our palate. Jeff Rubin points out, "In 1980, the US imported just over 40 percent of its fish. By 2005, it imported 70 percent. And . . . imported frozen lamb chops have gone from 10 percent of the US market in 1980 to over 40 percent twenty-five years later."[168] Nowhere is oil used more than in the business of producing the meat and dairy products we put on our table. Former cattle rancher Howard Lyman drives home this point in *Mad Cowboy*: "Energy is . . . required to control temperatures in the artificial 'living' environments of animals confined to feedlots, to transport feed to animals and to transport their waste away, to manufacture and transport antibiotics and other pharmaceuticals employed in the 'care' of animals in our animal factories."[169] A recent *New York Times* article also sheds light on the subject, citing the "enormous amounts of energy" consumed by the farming of livestock around the world:

> To put the energy-using demand of meat production into easy-to-understand terms, Gidon Eshel, a geophysicist at the Bard Center, and Pamela A. Martin, an assistant professor of geophysics at the University of Chicago, calculated that if Americans were to reduce meat consumption by just 20 percent it would be as if we all switched from a standard sedan—a Camry, say—to the ultra-efficient Prius. Similarly, a study last year by the National Institute of Livestock and Grassland Science in Japan estimated that 2.2 pounds of beef is responsible for the equivalent amount of carbon dioxide emitted by the average European car every 155 miles, and burns enough energy to light a 100-watt bulb for nearly 20 days.[170]

The UN Food and Agricultural Organization lists the following fossil fuel–consuming categories in the animal-foods industry:

1. Feed production. Fossil energy is used for the production of feeds, including land preparation, fertilizers, pesticides, harvesting, drying, and so on. It also includes their bulk transport (rail and/or sea freight), storage, processing, and distribution to the individual farms.
2. Farming operations. Once on the farm, and depending on location, season of the year, and building facilities, more fossil energy is needed for the movement of feeds from storage to the animal pens, for control of the thermal environment, and for animal waste collection and treatment.
3. Intermediate distribution. More fossil energy is required for the transport of products (meat animals to abattoirs, milk to processing plants, eggs to storage), processing (slaughtering,

pasteurization, manufacture of dairy products), storage, and refrigeration during transportation.
4. Final distribution and cooking. The distribution to the consumer and the final cooking process also require expenditures of fossil fuels.[171]

Did you know that it takes two calories of fossil fuel to produce one calorie of energy from soybeans? That doesn't sound like a very good deal until you learn that it takes fifty-four calories of fossil fuel to produce one calorie of energy from beef.[172] Herein lies a golden opportunity—perhaps the overall best opportunity to greatly reduce our global consumption of energy. On average, about twenty times more energy is required to produce meat calories than to produce whole-plant calories. According to an Ohio State University study, even the least efficient plant food is nearly ten times as efficient as the most efficient animal food.[173] Using the more conservative number from the study, we realize that we can produce plant calories with 90 percent less energy from fossil fuels than it takes to produce the same number of meat calories.

If we began a steady shift toward more plant-based foods, how big of a dent could we make in the consumption of fossil fuels? According to the Environmental Defense Fund (EDF), the animal-foods industry accounts for a whopping one-third of all fossil fuels consumed in the United States.[174] Let's do the math with these numbers. If we could save 90 percent of that one-third of our energy consumption, we could potentially reduce our total consumption of fossil fuel by 30 percent. Although some may challenge the numbers from the EDF, the fact remains that the production of animal-based foods is a highly inefficient process for deriving food calories for humans. Further, reducing our demand for products of this energy-consuming industry represents the world's only feasible near-term opportunity for making significant cuts in the global consumption of oil and other fossil fuels.

Peak Oil: When Will It Happen?

Like global warming, peak oil is a controversial topic. Scientists, economists, and oil people have been talking about it for a long time. The common definition of peak oil is the point in time when the highest rate of petroleum extraction is reached, after which the rate will never rise to the same volume again. Some reputable professionals believe that the world production of oil may have already peaked or will peak by 2015. Others argue that we will not reach that peak until 2030, 2050, or even later. Virtually all experts agree that the production of oil will peak eventually and then gradually decline over the course of this century. The only debate is when.

M. King Hubbert first modeled the concept of peak oil in 1956 to accurately predict that United States oil production would peak between 1965 and 1970. His logistic model, now called Hubbert peak theory, and its variants have described with reasonable accuracy the peak and decline of production from oil wells, fields, regions, and countries.

And while few believed him and many ridiculed him at the time, it turns out that Hubbert was pretty much on target as the U.S. production did peak in 1971 and has been in steady decline ever since—even with the expanding Alaskan oil that didn't peak until 1988 as you can see in the chart below. But when will we reach peak oil for the entire world?

According to Wikipedia on 7-18-2011, the optimists believe that peak oil won't happen until 2020 or later; whereas the pessimists think that it is happening now. Hubbert, who died in 1989, would have been among the pessimists. In whichever case, we know that oil is a finite resource and that our world will change dramatically when those limited quantities start driving the prices skyward.

Figure 5.1 is an example of a Hubbert curve for Alaska, clearly showing a peak followed by a steady decline. Notice that production grew steadily for twelve years from 1976 to 1988, when it hit its peak at just over 2 million barrels per day. It has declined steadily ever since, dipping below 1 million barrels per day in 2000 on its way to around 700,000 barrels in 2008. Production will decrease until the oil is totally depleted or it is no longer economically feasible to remove it from the ground. Every country is made of regions, oil fields, and individual wells. Every well eventually reaches a peak production level and begins to decline. The peak for a country, region, or field is reached when the sum total production of all of its wells begins to decline. Over fifty of the world's nations have reached their peak; only a handful remain that have not.

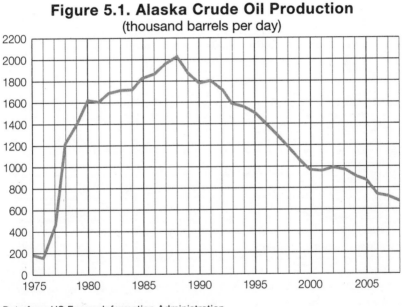

Figure 5.1. Alaska Crude Oil Production
(thousand barrels per day)

Data from US Energy Information Administration

Figure 5.1 Illustrating "peak oil" in one major oil-producing region of the world. Alaska crude oil production (in thousands of barrels per day)[175]

As you can see from Figure 5.2, our use of oil didn't really get into gear until the early 1900s. The chart takes various forecasts and assumptions into account and predicts that, with a demand curve of

2 percent per year, we will reach peak oil somewhere between 2026 and 2047. Keep in mind that some experts feel we may be at the peak oil stage right now and that when prices spike during the next expansion of the economy, they may not ever come back down to more reasonable levels. Remember when the price of oil reached $4.00 at the gas pump in May 2008? And again in April of 2011? The Great Recession tamped down the bubble for a few years, but the price is destined to continue its upward climb. If we have reached peak oil by the time of the next major expansion, $4.00 a gallon may sound like a bargain.

Figure 5.2. Annual Production Scenarios with 2 Percent Growth Rates and Different Resource Levels (Decline R/P=10)

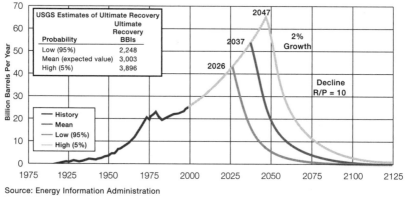

Source: Energy Information Administration
Note: U.S. volumes were added to the USGS foreign volumes to obtain world totals.

Figure 5.2 Annual production scenarios with 2 percent growth rates and different resource levels. Note: U.S. volumes were added to the USGS foreign volumes to obtain world totals.[176]

Biofuels to the Rescue?

Some may ask, "What about ethanol? Why can't ethanol help us post-pone that peak of our oil production?" Ethanol is one of those prom-ises that at first sounded almost too good to be true. But that was before we understood what was involved. The government got the ball rolling by offering some hefty incentives (a forty-five-cent-per-gallon tax credit) for ethanol use and production that promptly drove up the price of corn and dipped into taxpayers' pockets to the tune of $6 billion in 2009. On top of that, Americans pay another surcharge in the form of higher food prices. Jeff Rubin explains, "As more and more acres are converted to the production of corn, fewer and fewer acres are available for other crops that compete for the same land use. Soon the price of these other crops starts to rise as well."[177] The Congressional Budget Office, according to the *Wall Street Journal*, "estimates that from April 2007 to April 2008, 'the increased use of ethanol accounted for about 10 percent to 15 percent of the rise in food prices.'"[178] It has also meant higher food prices in other devel-oped countries. So far, ethanol production has created higher-priced corn followed by higher-priced food in general. What next?

It turns out that ethanol is no bargain for the environment either. The *Wall Street Journal* also cited a second study, by the Environmental Protection Agency's Office of Transportation and Air Quality, which "explains that the reduction in CO2 emissions from burning ethanol are minimal and maybe negative. Making ethanol requires new land from clearing forest and grasslands that would otherwise sequester carbon emissions."[179] Citing a UN study in October 2008, the *New York Times* reported, "[A] host of studies in the past year concluded that the rush to biofuels had some disastrous, if unintended, conse-quences for food security and the environment. Less food is available to eat in poor countries, global grain prices have skyrocketed and pre-cious forests have been lost as farmers have created fields to join the biofuel boom."[180]

It should be mentioned that U.S. agribusiness also persuaded the government to impose a fifty-four-cent tariff on every gallon of ethanol imported from Brazil, the world's second-largest maker of biofuels. Coincidentally, many experts consider Brazil's use of sugarcane stalks not only more efficient but better for the environment. The *Times* article elaborates on this point: "Worse still, specialists say, so much energy is required to convert many plants into fuel that the process does not result in a savings of carbon emissions. The OECD's report said only two food-based fuels were clearly environmentally better than fossil fuels when considering the entire 'life cycle' of their production: used cooking oil and sugar cane from Brazil. Sugar cane is far easier to convert to biofuel than most other crops."[181] So the U.S. tariff on Brazil's ethanol is protecting our own corn farmers at the expense of the environment.

Australian journalist Julian Cribb, in his investigation of the subject, sheds further light on the questionable strategy of replacing fossil fuels with ethanol. "Most current biofuels are not economically viable without subsidies: indeed, demand for them would collapse if they were priced at their real cost of production. According to various estimates, the United States props up its domestic ethanol industry with more than two hundred measures collectively costing taxpayers from six to twelve billion dollars a year, equivalent to a subsidy of thirty to one hundred cents on every liter sold."[182]

The huge incentives, as could be expected, have upset other agribusiness giants, because farmers are selling their corn to ethanol producers rather than to another primary customer—factory farms. Jeff Rubin writes of this problem of supply and demand: "If we continue to [increase ethanol production], corn will no longer be available as a food source for either humans or livestock. We will be taking food off the table to feed our cars."[183] Indeed, the price of corn soared in 2006 until farmers started producing more—at the expense of other products. The American Meat Institute (AMI) has been railing against ethanol for quite some time, including through an ad campaign on

Capitol Hill in April 2010 that left the National Corn Growers Association criticizing the AMI for "waging war" on ethanol and corn farmers.

The bottom line is that we clearly cannot depend on biofuels to solve our future energy problems. Not only have they ultimately driven up the price of food while costing taxpayers money, they are apparently causing even more problems for the environment. We'll have to find a more sustainable solution.

Timing Is Everything

Someday, future generations of the world's scientists will develop energy sources that will replace oil and the other fossil fuels. Those fuels may not be as cheap as oil has been, and we may not be able to enjoy for much longer the globe-trotting lifestyle that began in the twentieth century, but life will go on. After the hundred-year era of cheap oil, we'll have to transition to a completely different lifestyle. And we need time to smoothly make that transition—ideally enough time to avoid the riots, wars, and famine that could accompany an abrupt upsurge in the cost of oil.

We can hope this new energy of the future won't take too long to develop. But if we consider our progress in replacing fossil fuels so far, we could be looking at some pretty difficult times ahead. As for now, nuclear and renewable sources of energy such as geothermal, solar, wind, tide, and wave energy are providing a very small slice of the total pie. All renewable sources and nuclear power combined are only expected to contribute about 8 percent of the total energy mix by 2020. The International Energy Agency's Clean Energy report for 2011 projects that the nuclear share of the mix will actually drop to 5 percent by 2020, and the renewable group will grow to only 3 percent of the total.

But all is not doom and gloom. Many positives could result from the human race learning to get by on a fraction of the oil that it has been using during the early years of the twenty-first century. Less consumption of oil means less environmental damage and a change of lifestyle for many in the Western world—a lifestyle that features more dense living than many of the wealthier nations experience now. Europeans have been living with expensive oil for many years, and as a result, they have more efficient vehicles, smaller houses, denser neighborhoods, and a much greater use of mass transit. While the transition might be painful for some, the end result will likely be a better overall quality of life. To better understand what that might mean, ask yourself this question: where would you rather spend your vacation—Paris or Houston?

Further good news for Europe and the United States is that expensive oil means that the sprawling suburbs of the past will eventually be replaced by small farms, providing nearby residents with fresh, locally grown produce. Jeff Rubin explains, "During the 1990s, the American economy lost two acres of farmland every minute. Tomorrow's farm sector may be regaining those acres at the same pace."[184] And Bill McKibben sees a big environmental upside in such a development: "A Japanese study found that eating local food would be the equivalent of cutting household energy use by 20 percent."[185] Long range, life will be better in many ways—albeit much different. People will be working closer to home and will have more time to spend with their families or attend cultural or educational events.

Again, timing is everything in the completely connected global economy of the twenty-first century. Everyone remembers the pervasive fear that gripped the world during the devastating financial crisis of 2008. It's not too difficult to imagine what might happen if the price of gasoline soared to $10 a gallon but went down to only $7 or $8 with the next recession. Clearly, any industry that depends on transportation would suffer mightily—including airlines, hotels, retail, auto companies, and food. While this price increase wouldn't be too big of a jolt for densely populated Europe, it could be a disaster for millions of families in the United States.

Consider a middle-class family of five living on a cul-de-sac in the suburbs. With three or four drivers in the family, their monthly gasoline bill just went up several hundred dollars, followed shortly by sharp increases in their heating and electric bill. Many people in that situation might then decide to move into a smaller house near public transportation and closer to jobs, schools, and retail stores. As more people have the same idea, suddenly the home prices in the sprawling suburbs would begin to tumble. And, as we saw in 2008 and 2009, they don't have to tumble very far for people to start walking away from their homes—and their mortgages. When that starts happening, the economic downturn could go from bad to worse very quickly.

The simple answer to these problems is to use less energy—and to begin that process in earnest *now*. Switching to smaller, more efficient cars and homes and more densely populated communities connected by mass transit in a country like the United States will take time—lots of time—measured in decades, not in years. But everyone could take one step right away and save up to 30 percent of our total fossil fuel consumption. The single most powerful change you can make is to move as close as you can to a diet composed primarily of whole, plant-based foods. This collective action by enough people would provide us with time to learn how to live in a world without cheap oil—before it's too late.

"It is no use saying, 'We are doing our best.' You have got to succeed in doing what is necessary."

—Winston Churchill

6

MOUTHS TO FEED

"A hungry man is not a free man."

—Adlai Stevenson

L iving in a small coastal community in Connecticut, I understand the meaning of the phrase "It takes a village." The quality of life for everyone is enhanced by the interests and actions
of their neighbors; the whole can be greater than the sum of the parts.
Located on a densely populated peninsula, my quaint New England
village is almost like a small college campus where everyone eventually
gets to know one another.

Let's imagine that our village of 1,000 residents has 1,000 acres
of arable land within walking distance. The citizens and their leaders
must decide what to produce on that land: grain, cows, vegetables,
chickens, fruit, and/or pigs? If they proceed according to the model
in the world of today, they will use over 900 acres to produce lots of
meat and dairy products for the 300 wealthiest residents. That will
leave fewer than 100 acres to provide food for the remaining 700
people—clearly not enough land to survive, no matter what kind of

food they are eating. Sounds absurd, right? But that is the direction we are headed in the early part of the twenty-first century.

The world's model for feeding all her people has sprung a few leaks. As with oil and with fresh water, we are beginning to find that arable land is a finite resource. This problem, combined with the crises discussed in the previous two chapters on the environment and energy, points to the likelihood of much more world hunger in our future, not less. To summarize:

- The world population continues to grow, mainly in the developing world.
- Millions more are adopting the inefficient Western diet each year.
- The arable land available for farming grows smaller every day.
- More demand for food on less land drives prices higher.
- Future water shortages will limit productivity for all.
- The next rise in energy prices will exacerbate all of the above.

Something has to give. With the world's population projected to reach 9 billion by 2050, we're in for some serious price hikes in food unless the balance in what we eat changes soon. Clearly, the path we're taking is not going to work in the future. The obvious solution would be a planned, systematic shift in the direction of consuming primarily plant-based food, but the reverse is happening. Millions of people in the developing world who grew up eating plants are now rushing to buy animal-based foods as soon as they can afford them.

As Julian Cribb explains in *The Coming Famine*, "The first thing people do as they climb out of poverty is to improve their diet. Demand for protein foods such as meat, milk, fish, and eggs from consumers with better incomes, mainly in India and China but also in Southeast Asia and Latin America, is rising rapidly. This in turn requires vastly more grain to feed the animals and fish."[186] As a person comes out of poverty, he naturally feels that "improving" his diet means copying what the wealthier people have been eating for a long time. Eric

Schlosser in *Fast Food Nation* provides another reason for the adoption of this new diet: "The anthropologist Yunxiang Yan has noted that in the eyes of Beijing consumers, McDonald's represents 'Americana and the promise of modernization.'"[187] Little do they know that while they may begin to crave the calorie-dense foods, "improvement" in terms of their health is not part of the bargain, and neither is their continued ability to be able to afford the "rich" foods they have recently learned to love.

The Poor Won't Go Quietly

The problem of food shortages is not just a hypothetical threat looming in the hazy future. Already the rich Western diet has negatively affected the poor. While the developed world was focused on the financial crisis that struck in 2008, many starving people of the world were stirred by a more basic fear: how to put food on the table.

World farm commodity prices skyrocketed almost 70 percent during 2007 and the first half of 2008. According to a February 2008 article in the *Guardian*, the UN's World Food Programme officials say "the extraordinary increases in the global price of basic foods were caused by a 'perfect storm' of factors: a rise in demand for animal feed from increasingly prosperous populations in India and China, the use of more land and agricultural produce for biofuels, and climate change. The impact has been felt around the world. Food riots have broken out in Morocco, Yemen, Mexico, Guinea, Mauritania, Senegal and Uzbekistan."[188] Note that Mexico, a prime beneficiary of the farming technology initiatives of the Green Revolution, is included in that list.

And the economic downturn of 2008 was hardly the only event to trigger a food crisis. The effect that one bad harvest for a major food exporter can have on the world's food supply was amply shown after an unprecedented number of forest fires reduced Russia's 2010 harvest so much that it shut off all food exports. The *New York Times* reported one immediate repercussion: "Food prices rose 5 percent globally during August, according to the United Nations, spurred mostly by the higher cost of wheat, and the first signs of unrest erupted as 10 people died in Mozambique during clashes ignited partly by a 30 percent leap in the cost of bread."[189] The world is a village indeed. As you can see from the headlines in the box, world hunger is nothing new, and the leaders of our global village have been talking about this topic for a long time. Even when there has been plenty of land, water, and energy available for growing food, hunger has been an issue for the poorest people in the world. But if the leaders of the past couldn't solve the problem without the shortage of natural resources that we face today, how can we expect today's leaders to solve it now?

A SAMPLING OF HISTORICAL HEADLINES

New York Times, October 14, 1945
WORLD HUNGER PUT AS CAUSE OF WARS
Secretary Anderson Hopes the Coming Meeting of UNFAO
Will Solve Food Problems

New York Times, November 11, 1958
Eisenhower Asks Crusade on World Hunger, Disease
Outlines a Program to Colombo Meeting for Expansion of Trade
With and Aid to the Under-Developed Lands

New York Times, February 4, 1978
Administration Plans to Set Up Commission on World Hunger
President Carter intends to establish a Commission on World Hunger

---

To be sure, the prospect of solving this problem anytime soon with current methods seems more remote than ever. The situation has become urgent and requires immediate action. Jean Ziegler, vice president of the UN Human Rights Council Advisory Committee, made the following appeal to world leaders in January 2010: "In a world overflowing with riches, it is an outrageous scandal that more than 1 billion people suffer from hunger and malnutrition and that every year over 6 million children die of starvation and related causes. We must take urgent action now."[190]

A Little Background

Hunger is more than simply not getting enough calories; it also involves nutrient deficiencies, which take many lives. Providing the hard numbers, Ziegler reported in 2006 that mortality from malnutrition accounted for 58 percent of the world's total mortality. "In the world, approximately 62 million people, all causes of death combined, die each year . . . In 2006, more than 36 million died of hunger or diseases due to deficiencies in micronutrients."[191] That computes to almost 100,000 people per day—that's two people for every word in this book *every day*. Further, the World Health Organization reports that 3.7 billion people of the world's current total of 6.7 billion are malnourished—the largest number of malnourished people in history.[192]

The need for more food production was recognized as far back as the end of World War II. Even then, agricultural experts realized that the amount of arable land could not be increased dramatically, so scientists concentrated on improving crop yield instead. This movement led to what is known as the Green Revolution. A jump in production occurred after new hybrid strains were developed for such major crops as wheat, rice, and corn. These hardier varieties were introduced into developing countries during the 1960s and 1970s, along with a new emphasis on chemical fertilizers and irrigation.

The first major leap was the breeding of a dwarf strain of wheat by U.S. agronomist Norman Borlaug, winner of the Nobel Peace Prize in 1970. When this strain was introduced into Mexico, it resulted in a doubling of the country's wheat crop. When famine threatened in India and Pakistan in the 1960s, Borlaug's new methods nearly doubled Pakistan's wheat yield between 1965 and 1970 and increased India's "from 12.3 million tons of wheat in 1965 to 20 million tons in 1970."[193] Equally revolutionary was the development by the International Rice Research Institute of a new variety of rice that would grow even when submerged in three feet of water. After it was introduced in the Philippines, the new hybrid produced five times as much rice as the country was producing before. In addition, its hardiness meant many new acres prone to seasonal flooding could be used for crop production.

These kinds of gains were encouraging at the time but have proven to be too little too late as the world's population continues to skyrocket. Since the 1970s, many of the initial gains of the Green Revolution have leveled off—dramatically in some cases. "For example, rice yields per acre in South Korea grew nearly 60 percent from 1961 to 1977, but only 1 percent from 1977 to 2000. Rice production in Asia as a whole grew an average of 3.2 percent per year from 1967 to 1984 but only 1.5 percent per year from 1984 to 1996."[194] The problem is that the population is growing at a much higher rate, and the percentage of those eating a meat-based diet is expected to rise from 33 to 40 percent by 2050. Where is the difference going to be made up? The problem is exacerbated by the fact that many farmers in developing countries have depleted their water resources in irrigating their crops, as noted in Chapter 4. This means that dramatic new improvements will likely not be found within the same amount of acreage.

An Unsustainable Model for Feeding People

No matter what level of humanitarian concern for the world's poorest people exists, with the dynamics in place today, the situation is likely to get much worse before it gets better. The combination of more people, higher energy costs, and a shortage of arable land points to the fact that our feeding model is not going to get the job done in the future.

Let's take a look at our current model for the Western world—the same one that's rapidly being adopted in the developing world. By cycling our grain through livestock, we waste 90 percent of its protein, 96 percent of its calories, 100 percent of its fiber, and 100 percent of its carbohydrates.[195] Further, to feed a single person the typical Western diet (heavy with animal products) for a year requires 3.25 acres of arable land. To feed one vegan requires about one-sixth of an acre.[196] Thus, with the vegan diet, you can feed about twenty people with the same amount of land that is required to feed one person with the typical Western diet. As of July 2010, the U.S. Census reports that the total world population is 6.85 billion people;[197] the FAO reports that there are 4.2 billion acres of arable land.[198] This means there are 1.15 acres theoretically available to grow food for each human being on the planet today. What's wrong with this picture? If we have just over one acre of available arable land per person, it is obvious that everyone cannot eat the rich Western diet. There simply isn't enough land.

Mark Bittman emphasizes this point in his *New York Times* book review of *The Coming Famine*: "Mr. Cribb is reporting on the fate of a planet whose resources have, in the last 200 years, been carelessly, even ruthlessly exploited for the benefit of the minority. Now that the majority is beginning to demand—or at least crave—the same kind of existence, it's clear that, population boom or not, there simply isn't enough of the Euro-American way of life to go around."[199]

In *Why Your World Is about to Get a Whole Lot Smaller*, Jeff Rubin reports on World Bank president Robert Zoellick's 2008 warning of a mounting "human crisis." He was referring to the millions of the world's poorest people who have been driven into malnutrition as a result of high food prices. "'While people in the developed world are focused on the financial crisis,' Zoellick said, 'many forget that a human crisis is rapidly unfolding in developing countries. It is pushing poor people to the brink of survival . . . There is only so much arable land on the planet. In fact, climate change may mean there is less of it all the time.'"[200]

The problem is made worse by the steady degradation of the world's arable land. Each year, the world loses over 24 million acres of arable land.[201] This is an area about the size of South Carolina. Causes are soil erosion, water shortages, climate issues, and deforestation. Most of this loss is attributable to the livestock industry, according to the 2006 UN Report *Livestock's Long Shadow*, covered extensively in Chapter 4. This steady loss needs to be evaluated against a steadily growing population. Both UN and U.S. officials now project that our population will continue to grow and will exceed 9 billion by 2050. For the past sixty years, our global population has increased by about 72 million people per year. That's 197,000 people per day—an amount equal to the entire population of Grand Rapids, Michigan!

And there's one more problem. Meat-based foods are also notoriously wasted by the wealthy, with up to one-third of the food simply spoiling before use or being thrown out because of expiration dates. One of the biggest problems with a meat-based diet is that meat spoils quickly, meaning that a great deal of this inefficiently produced food is simply thrown away. Julian Cribb points out the scale of the problem in Great Britain:

> A former government food advisor, Lord Haskins of Skidby, who worked for one of the nation's largest food suppliers, had calculated that 60 million Britons were each year wasting around 20 million tonnes [22 million U.S. tons] of food—16 million tonnes in homes, shops, supermarkets, wholesalers, markets, and manufacturing establishments, and around 4 million tonnes on the farm or in transit. The average household could save $1,000 a year on

food purchases if even a fifth of this wastage could be eliminated. The chief culprit, it turned out, was the use-by date, which was causing consumers to throw out one-third of all the food they bought.[202]

To summarize, we have more people, less arable land, more land required per person, and excessive spoilage and waste. As more of the world continues to move in the direction of the rich Western diet, the average acreage of land required per person will continue to grow, and that simply can't be accommodated. We have two choices. We either dramatically reduce the number of people on the planet (not so easy), or we start an immediate movement toward a global feeding model that maximizes the consumable calories from each acre of land. If enough people consumed a land-, water-, and energy-efficient plant-based diet, we could easily feed the world's future population on far less than half of the 7.9 billion acres of arable land available. As an added bonus, we would free up billions of acres that are currently used for growing food for humans and their animals, and that land could be returned to forests and other natural habitats and put to work restoring the biodiversity and ecological balance that has been slipping away for the past fifty years.

Our Feeding Model Will Change Eventually

In a world where the human population continues to add another Grand Rapids every day, a South Carolina–sized chunk of arable land is lost each year, and the developing countries steadily move toward a highly inefficient meat-based diet, we simply must start addressing the root causes of a rapidly approaching global feeding crisis. The first step is sharing the information with everyone. For many people, world hunger has always been out of sight and out of mind. The average citizen of the Western world has no idea of the global consequences of what he has chosen to put on his plate.

Once enough people understand the "big picture" of how every- thing we've discussed fits together, a take-charge minority will begin making changes in their own lives and will continue to spread the word. They will form the first wave of the grassroots revolution that will inevitably lead to some big changes in the way we feed the human population of the world. Eventually, when a sufficiently large number of people join this movement, the world's top leaders will have enough political support to make this effort public policy.

But for now, a grassroots mandate for change must be led by people like you and me—the informed minority who understands the gravity of what is at stake. Someone asked me recently, "Will our changing to a plant-based diet really do any good for the hungry? Or is this kind of like your parents saying that you must clean your plate because people are starving in China?" No, it's not like that at all. Simple math shows that our current food model cannot possibly continue to feed the world. But the good news is that every person who chooses to replace the animal products on his or her plate with plant-based foods will personally free up several acres of arable land—enough land to feed another fifteen or twenty people.

When it comes to taking care of our environment and efficiently feeding our growing human population, our current feeding model is not going to survive for very much longer. As reported in the previ- ously mentioned movie, *HOME*, "In just the last 50 years, humankind has inflicted more damage on the fragile harmony of nature than all the previous generations of humans combined for the past 200,000 years." And much of that damage is directly related to how we have chosen to eat in the western world—a harmful, wasteful, and grossly unsustainable diet-style that (per calorie) requires 20 times more land, 20 times more fossil fuel energy, and 20 times more water than does the natural diet for our species—whole, plant-based foods.

Sometimes it's painful to learn the truth about such a crucial issue. You almost yearn for the carefree days when you were ignorant about the dilemma. But now that you understand the big picture, perhaps the joy of taking action and making a difference in this tragic problem will replace the pleasure of eating the unhealthy foods of your past.

"Human rights rest on human dignity. The dignity of man is an ideal worth fighting for and worth dying for."

—Robert Maynard

7

HELL ON EARTH

"Teaching a child not to step on a caterpillar is as valuable
to the child as it is to the caterpillar."

—Bradley Millar

The chickens, pigs, cows, and sheep of my youth appeared to
have a pretty nice life—at least up until the last day of it. What
happened to that picture? In short, the raising of those animals
for our dinner tables has become a very big business.

In a free market system, all businesses exert a constant push to
increase sales, lower costs, gain market share, and make more money.
While millions of small farms around the country once provided local
markets with meat and dairy products, now just a handful of gigantic
corporations control our food supply. Those companies do not regard
the animals we eat as living and breathing beings—they are units of
production. They are raised in strict uniformity to produce the largest
animal in the shortest amount of time. They are housed in an environment that has become known as the factory farm, technically called a
contained animal feeding operation (CAFO). Many people have heard
about them, but only a tiny percentage of the population has seen the

inside of one. That's exactly how the industry would like to keep it. As Paul McCartney has commented, "If slaughterhouses had glass walls, everyone would be a vegetarian."

Books and magazine articles have been written about the horrors of the modern-day factory farm, specials have aired on television, and videos are available on the internet. We all know vaguely what is going on, but most of us don't wish to think about it. We'd prefer to keep rationalizing that we "need that protein," and the more committed of us try to buy free-range chicken, grass-fed beef, or wild fish. At the same time, we find the Michael Vick dog-fighting saga utterly despicable. So do we really care about animals or not? Jonathan Foer describes our somewhat odd situation very well in *Eating Animals*: "When surveyed, 96 percent of Americans say that animals deserve legal protection, 76 percent say that animal welfare is more important to them than low meat prices, and nearly two-thirds advocate passing not only laws but 'strict laws' concerning the treatment of farmed animals. You'd be hard-pressed to find any other issue on which so many people see eye to eye."[203]

Part of the reason many people turn a blind eye is that they are not fully aware how animals raised for food actually live. We imagine in our mind's eye a rural idyll out of a Currier and Ives print. The reality is quite different. David Kirby in *Animal Factory* points out the contrast: "Structures that house poultry and livestock are sometimes called parlors or barns—though they bear no resemblance to the quaint red structures with haylofts that are so iconic to American country life. CAFO houses are usually massive, hangarlike structures made of concrete and aluminum or heavy canvas. In some megadairies, they are a quarter-mile long."[204]

Occasionally, a newspaper will feature one of these operations, usually after what has become a recurring problem in our food supply: infection spread from animals to humans. Recently, after 1,500 cases of salmonella poisoning were reported, one of the most notorious factory farms in the United States had to recall a half billion eggs. "Barns

infested with flies, maggots and scurrying rodents, and overflowing
manure pits were among the widespread food safety problems that
federal inspectors found at a group of Iowa egg farms at the heart
of a nationwide recall and salmonella outbreak," reported the *New
York Times* in August 2010. Michael R. Taylor, deputy commissioner
for food for the FDA, declared that "in response to the outbreak and
recall, F.D.A. inspectors would visit all of the 600 major egg-producing
facilities in the country over the next 15 months. Those farms, with
50,000 or more hens each, represent about 80 percent of nationwide
egg production."[205]

Many other incidents of a similar nature have occurred, but rather
than dwell on yesterday's headlines, this chapter focuses on the animals
that are the hosts of such diseases. John Robbins devoted entire chapters to each of these animals in his best-selling book *Diet for a New
America* in 1987. Unfortunately, even though the big food producers
would disagree, things have become worse for the animals since then.
Why? In 1987, there were thousands of small farms producing a good
portion of the meat, milk, and eggs in the United States and other Western countries. Today, only an estimated 1 percent of our animal-based
foods are produced on farms where the farmer-owners still care about
the quality of life for the animals involved. Let's take a look at how our
eggs, chicken, hamburgers, sausage, and shrimp are produced.

Chicken Feed

Sometimes as little children, we would get baby chickens in our Easter
baskets. There is probably not a cuter, move loveable animal in the
world than a baby chick. They strut around full of life, chirping, and
simply enjoying their new world outside the egg. But whether female
or male, over 99 percent of the newborn chicks of today are in for a
life of misery followed by a horrible death.

Best-selling author and journalist Michael Pollan describes the lives of the female chickens in egg factories: "It is routine practice to cram laying hens into cages so small that the birds are sometimes driven to cannibalize their cagemates. The solution to this 'vice'—as the industry and the Department of Agriculture call such counterproductive behaviors in livestock (talk about blaming the victims!)—is to snip the beaks off the hens with hot knives, without the use of anesthetic."[206]

Although European authorities have taken more vigorous action to enforce anticruelty standards, Jane Goodall describes a similarly Dickensian picture in England:

> Much of our poultry is raised in "battery farms," buildings in which hundreds of cages are stacked one on top of the other. In battery farms with laying hens, a single shed may contain up to 70,000 caged birds. The hens are crammed four or even six together, into small wire cages, so close they cannot stretch their wings. Because they then tend to peck one another, their beaks are often "trimmed" in a painful de-beaking process. And because their claws frequently get caught in the wire mesh on the floor of their cages, they are sometimes trimmed by cutting off the end of the toes so that they cannot grow again.[207]

John Robbins offers a human analogy of the misery: "[P]icture yourself standing in a crowded elevator. The elevator is so crowded, in fact, that your body is in contact on all sides with other bodies. Even to turn around in place would be difficult. And one more thing to keep in mind—this is your life. It is not just a temporary bother, until you get to your floor. This is permanent. Your only release will be at the hands of the executioner."[208]

In addition to these deplorable conditions, the laying hen must also endure food and light deprivation—a modern technique for generating more eggs per bird. "Factory farms commonly manipulate food and light to increase productivity, often at the expense of the animals' welfare. Egg farmers do this to reboot birds' internal clocks so they start laying valuable eggs faster and, crucially, at the same time."[209] As one farmer explains in *Eating Animals*, common practice is to keep the hens in darkness for a while on almost a starvation diet and then turn on the lights almost full time to trick them into thinking it's springtime, when their internal clock tells them it's time to start laying again.[210]

MOVEABLE FEASTS

The suffering of animals does not end at the factory farm. Those animals that must be transported to slaughterhouses are subjected to a new form of compacting. The Humane Society of the United States reveals this part of the sad cycle: "Billions of farm animals endure the rigors of transport each year in the United States, with millions of pigs, cows, and 'spent' egg-laying hens traveling across the country. Overcrowded onto trucks that do not provide any protection from temperature extremes, animals travel long distances without food, water, or rest. The conditions are so stressful that in-transit death is considered common."[211] As awful as the procedures on egg-laying factory farms are, chickens raised for human consumption face in some ways a worse fate. The first problem is how they are force-fed. The Humane Society of the United States has reported: "The chicken industry's selective breeding for fast-growing animals and use of growth-promoting antibiotics have produced birds whose bodies struggle to function and are on the verge of structural collapse. To put this growth rate into perspective, the University of Arkansas reports that if humans grew as fast as today's chickens, we'd weigh 349 pounds by our second birthday."[212]

If you think the females in an egg factory have it bad, consider what happens to their brothers. Since they are not genetically designed to produce meat and obviously wouldn't be able to cut it as a laying hen, they are simply destroyed. How many? Half of all the baby chicks born in egg factories each year—more than 250 million—are male, and that's just in the United States.[213] How are they destroyed? "Most male layers are destroyed by being sucked through a series of pipes onto an electrified plate. Other layer chicks are destroyed in other ways, and it's impossible to call those animals more or less fortunate. Some are tossed into large plastic containers. The weak are trampled to the bottom, where they suffocate slowly. The strong suffocate slowly at the top. Others are sent fully conscious through macerators (picture a wood chipper filled with chicks)."[214] All of this torture takes place at the hands of humans without the slightest acknowledgment that these are living, sentient beings.

As for the broiler chickens, when they are overstuffed enough, they endure an equally miserable end. "At the slaughter plant, birds are moved off trucks, dumped from transport crates onto conveyors, and hung upside down by their legs in shackles. Their heads pass through electrified baths of water, intended to immobilize them before their throats are slit. From beginning to end, the entire process is filled with pain and suffering."[215]

The *New York Times* reported recently that several of the major producers of chickens destined for our white supermarket bins have invented a more humane treatment: "Two premium chicken producers, Bell & Evans in Pennsylvania and Mary's Chickens in California, are preparing to switch to a system of killing their birds that they consider more humane. The new system uses carbon dioxide gas to gently render the birds unconscious before they are hung by their feet to have their throats slit."[216] Perhaps it is an improvement, but it raises an interesting question: in what sort of world is the gas chamber a step up?

Happy Meals for the Kids

Even more so than "mom and apple pie," these days the best short descriptor of the American way of life is "burger and fries." From the time a child is old enough to talk, she is old enough for her first hamburger. And she may actually grow up thinking that hamburgers are one of the four major food groups—the others being chicken nuggets, grilled cheese, and fish and chips. (Anyone wondering why millions of kids are obese these days?) So let's take a look at a day or two in the miserable life of a baby hamburger.

Some people who have been there report that life is better (ever so slightly) for cows than for the animals in the pig and chicken CAFOs of the world. Don't try telling that to the newborn male calf. Shortly after being separated from his mother and her milk for life, he is castrated. According to an article on TheBeefSite.com, castration is recommended to reduce meat toughness and minimize aggressive behavior in the animals. The suggested age is shortly after birth.[217] Keep in mind that a baby calf, unlike a human newborn, is walking around and very much aware of his surroundings just hours after birth. Castration without the use of an anesthetic is an almost universal practice, even in the most humane of cattle farms. After that introduction to the world, do you think that calf would be surprised to know that he will someday become a Happy Meal?

While not quite as cramped and uncomfortable as the laying hen, the average beef cow spends his life in miserable confinement until he reaches the ripe old age of eighteen months, when he is ready for slaughter. Eric Schlosser in *Fast Food Nation* supplies some of the particulars:

> The ConAgra Beef Company runs the nation's biggest meatpacking complex . . . To supply the beef slaughterhouse, ConAgra operates a pair of enormous feedlots. Each of them can hold up to one hundred thousand head of cattle. At times the animals are crowded so closely together it looks like a sea of cattle, a mooing, moving mass of brown and white fur that goes on for acres. These cattle don't eat blue grama and buffalo grass off the prairie. During the three months before slaughter, they eat grain dumped into long concrete troughs that resemble highway dividers. The grain fattens the cattle quickly, aided by the anabolic steroids implanted in their ear.[218]

The slaughter is a process that is closely shielded by the industry. As Michael Pollan describes, "[S]laughter [is the] one event in [my personally owned cow's] life I was not allowed to witness or even learn anything about, save its likely date. This didn't exactly surprise me: The meat industry understands that the more people know about what happens on the kill floor, the less meat they're likely to eat."[219] Jonathan Foer discovered the same guarded practices while spending three years researching for *Eating Animals.* "I couldn't get near the inside of a large slaughter facility," he reports. "Just about the only way for someone outside the industry to see industrial cattle slaughter is to go undercover, and that is not only a project that takes half a year or more, it can be life-threatening work."[220]

Even though the industry would prefer that no one ever see the inside of a slaughterhouse, occasionally it happens. Somehow, back in 2000, the San Francisco–based Humane Farming Association managed to get some very revealing videotape on television. Aired first by an NBC affiliate in Seattle and in 2001 by *Dateline NBC*, the videos were difficult to watch, but they accurately portrayed what was going on behind the scenes. "The tapes showed struggling cows hoisted upside down and butchered while still alive. Fully conscious cows were shown being skinned alive, their legs cut off while struggling for freedom. Cows were shown being hit repeatedly with stunning devices that didn't work. Other cows were tormented and repeatedly shocked with electric prods. And workers were shown shoving an electric prod into a cow's mouth."[221]

Such graphic scenes couldn't be further from the American myth of the cowboy herding cattle on the plains. They are a sad statement that modern practices are hardly better than the atrocities Upton Sinclair reported about the Chicago stockyards in *The Jungle*, written over a hundred years ago. Those big dumb beasts chewing their cud deserve a more peaceful fate than becoming tomorrow night's rib-eye steak.

Sausage on Your Pizza?

You've probably heard many people comment about not wanting to know all the ingredients that go into sausage. Well, you also don't want to know about the suffering of today's pigs during their part of the sausage-making process.

It should be pointed out first that pigs are fairly evolved animals, judged by scientists to have the intelligence of a three-year-old child. They are a much cleaner and more refined animal than their reputation would suggest. As John Robbins reports, "Pigs are highly social and active creatures, who will in a natural setting travel 30 miles a day grazing, rooting, and interacting with their environment. In the evening, groups of pigs will prepare a communal nest from branches and grass, in which they will spend the night together."[222] It was not by accident that George Orwell chose pigs to run the uprising in his famous novel *Animal Farm.*

The pig's life as a future pizza topping is not nearly as pleasant. David Kirby in *Animal Factory* describes their depressing life cycle:

[B]aby pigs are delivered from (usually) artificially inseminated sows that live much of their cramped lives in small "gestation crates" that afford them no room to stand up or turn around . . . After castration, the young boars are called barrows. These animals will never go outside, breathe fresh air, or feel natural sunlight. They will not get a chance to grub in dirt or wallow in mud, as pigs are meant to do . . . By the time the animals near market size, they are so large that they have to be packed into their small indoor pens. There is little room for them to move around. This often results in higher incidences of infectious diseases, bloody fights, and highly stressed animals with weakened immune systems. At about five months of age, the hogs are dispatched to the slaughterhouse.[223]

Jeff Tietz provides in his 2006 *Rolling Stone* article another vivid picture of a factory pig's confinement: "Forty fully grown 250-pound male hogs often occupy a pen the size of a tiny apartment. They trample each other to death. There is no sunlight, straw, fresh air or earth."[224] He goes on to discuss the multitude of health hazards that pigs face while they are being fattened up for slaughter:

> Taken together, the immobility, poisonous air and terror of confinement badly damage the pigs' immune systems. They become susceptible to infection, and in such dense quarters microbes or parasites or fungi, once established in one pig, will rush spritelike through the whole population. Accordingly, factory pigs are infused with a huge range of antibiotics and vaccines, and are doused with insecticides. Without these compounds—oxytetracycline, draxxin, ceftiofur, tiamulin—diseases would likely kill them.[225]

Shockingly, these barbaric practices are only the prelude to an ending that might make anybody swear off ever eating a holiday ham again. David Kirby followed these poor creatures all the way to their untimely demise. "In the slaughterhouse," he writes, "the assembly-line nature of CAFOs was made more vivid. Live pigs were shoved onto sharp hooks and dangled from an elevated conveyor belt. Workers shot them in the head with a bolt bullet and then, after they died, sliced open their bellies in a rush of blood and entrails. The living pigs waiting on hooks witnessed all of this."[226]

Catch of the Day

Many so-called vegetarians eat fish, at least once in a while. While the suffering of "real animals," with legs and lungs like we have, is better known, we don't hear a great deal about the suffering that humans have inflicted on the creatures with fins and gills. This takes place in two major areas: open-sea fishing and fish farms. It turns out that Charlie the Tuna is not quite as happy as StarKist wants us to believe.

Out on the open sea, the problems of overfishing have been known for a long time. The most famous example is the collapse of Atlantic cod fishing off the Grand Banks, but there are numerous other examples, such as the crash of anchovy fisheries off Peru or the near extinction of sole in the seas around Great Britain. China has now resorted to a total ban on fishing in the South China Sea for part of the year. As the world moves more toward eating fish as a substitute for meat, the problem has only grown worse.

An insidious by-product of ocean fishing is all the fish that are caught by accident, called bycatch. Bycatch is defined as sea creatures that are caught unintentionally while fishing for another species. The highest rates of bycatch are associated with shrimp trawlers. For every pound of shrimp that you find on that nicely arranged platter, roughly *twenty-six* pounds of other sea creatures were killed and thrown back into the ocean. Although it accounts for only 2 percent of the global seafood by weight, shrimp trawling accounts for 33 percent of the world's bycatch. As Jonathan Foer explains, "Trawling, almost always for shrimp, is the marine equivalent of clear-cutting rain forest. Whatever they target, trawlers sweep up fish, sharks, rays, crabs, squid, scallops—typically about a hundred different fish and other species. Virtually all die."[227]

Another method of catching healthy wild fish is to use the longline, a heavy fishing line that can be miles long and has many hooks at intervals. One study mentioned in *Eating Animals* found that "roughly 4.5 million sea animals are killed as bycatch in longline fishing every year, including roughly 3.3 million sharks, 1 million marlins, 60,000 sea turtles, 75,000 albatross, and 20,000 dolphins and whales."[228]

The drastic decline in world fisheries has led to the practice of fish farming. While this practice does save some fish out in the open ocean, fish farms create severe environmental problems. One problem is all the wild fish that are consumed by farmed species like shrimp, salmon, trout, bass, and yellowtail tuna. The ratio for salmon, the most common farmed fish, is three pounds of eaten fish to every pound of salmon. This ratio reaches as high as five pounds of wild ocean fish to produce a single pound of other farmed fish.[229]

The most prominent of the hazards is the waste the fish emit within their confined area offshore. Barry Estabrook comments in the *Atlantic*, "A salmon farm is nothing more than a vast, floating feedlot, except feedlots, at least nominally, have to dispose of food waste, dead animals, and excrement in suitable containment areas. Salmon feedlots flush it all into the sea."[230] According to an article in *Time*, this has led to serious contamination of coastal areas from Maine to Chile to Thailand, where "[l]ong strips of coastline south of Bangkok now look like powdery gray moonscapes."[231]

The fish being farmed face equally grave hazards. John Robbins reports, "Fish farming is one of the most intensive forms of animal agriculture. As many as 40,000 fish may be crammed into a cage, with each fish given the equivalent of half a bathtub of water in which to spend its life . . . In 1990, only 6 percent of the salmon consumed in the world were the product of fish farms. But by 1998, the number had risen to 40 percent."[232] Not surprisingly, conditions for the fish in fish farms aren't too different from the disgusting conditions experienced by their land-based counterparts. Foer also cites several of the atrocities that farmed fish must endure, including "water so fouled that it makes it hard to breathe [and] crowding so intense that animals begin to cannibalize one another."[233]

A Moral Dilemma for the Ages

Although the manner of killing animals for food has only lately reached its chilling industrial efficiency, some great thinkers have been talking about the need to end the practice of eating animals for centuries. Leonardo da Vinci spoke out about animals over 500 years ago, saying, "The time will come when men such as I will look on the murder of animals as they now look on the murder of men." Another highly respected citizen of his time, Thomas Alva Edison, also addressed our uncivilized treatment of animals. He said, "Nonviolence leads to the highest ethics, which is the goal of all evolution. Until we stop harming all other living beings, we are still savages."

Like many of those great thinkers of history, the vast majority of people today despise the mistreatment of animals. Yet we have turned a blind eye to the modern methods of putting food on our plates. Fortunately, the awareness continues to grow as these atrocities are revealed by mainstream authors and reporters. The following is from an article by Maggie Jones that appeared in 2008 in the *New York Times Magazine*.

It was an animal rights advocate's dream: Pacelle and his organization had shuttered this $100 million plant, the Westland/Hallmark Meat Company, with the help of an undercover investigator wearing a hidden video camera with a lens the size of the tip of a pen. Over six weeks last year, the investigator—a vegan who brought soy-riblet sandwiches for lunch—filmed workers using chains to drag cows too sick or too injured to stand. The workers jabbed cows with electrical prods and rolled them with a forklift to get them onto their feet and into the slaughter chute. In addition to being excessively cruel, it was a risk to human health: cows too sick or injured to walk are more vulnerable to E. coli, mad cow and other diseases.[234]

Michael Pollan addresses similar issues for other animals: "Mutilating pigs and chickens while they are alive is as routine in modern American agriculture as bacon and eggs for breakfast. These operations are performed every day on thousands of factory farms that are owned by, or under contract to, Fortune 500 corporations that supply hundreds of thousands of restaurants and supermarkets." He says of animal suffering in general, "The lives of billions of animals on American feedlots and factory farms are horrible to contemplate, an affront to our image of ourselves as humane . . . To peer over the increasingly high walls of our industrial animal agriculture is not only to lose your appetite but to feel revulsion and shame."[235] Jonathan Foer poses the really hard question that all of us must eventually answer: "Whether we're talking about fish species, pigs, or some other eaten animal, is such suffering the most important thing in the world? Obviously not. But that's not the question. Is it more important than sushi, bacon, or chicken nuggets? That's the question."[236]

If my father had written this book back when I was a child, he would not have included a chapter about the suffering of animals. Why not? Because in those days, farm animals just didn't suffer as much—certainly not when compared to the horrible level of suffering that pervades over 95 percent of the industry today. They lived a pretty good life and, in most cases, were truly loved and respected by their owners. The farmer of old knew that his animals needed to remain happy and healthy for him to be able to make a living—they were partners, in a sense.

But now the CAFOs of the world are raising some 60 billion animals (not counting fish) a year for our dinner tables. We now know that all those billions of animals are suffering constantly—every minute that they are alive—and their numbers continue to grow. While demand has leveled off in many of the OECD countries, the animal-based Western diet is just now beginning to explode in developing countries such as China and India. The potential future numbers are staggering. Says Foer, "If the world followed America's lead, it would consume over 165 billion chickens annually (even if the world population didn't increase)."[237] Do we really want to kill three times as many animals as we are killing now?

We know from surveys that over 95 percent of the people in the U.S. care about the treatment of animals. Yet we continue to support the atrocities taking place with every dollar we spend on animal-based foods. The horrors are out of sight and out of mind. There are now almost 7 billion humans on Earth, but there are nine times as many living, breathing animals that spend their entire lives each year in a *hell on Earth* for one reason only—so that we can enjoy the pleasure of eating their flesh. By simply voting with our food choices, we can end that hell once and for all.

The prospect of ending the worldwide suffering of animals raised for our dinner tables is an excellent reason to begin an aggressive shift to a plant-based diet. And as awareness grows, the issue will resonate with hundreds of millions of people throughout the world. But if this isn't enough reason, remember the other four compelling reasons to make the switch: human health and the unsustainable cost of healthcare, the fragile environment, the looming energy crisis, and world hunger. We must take decisive steps before we leave Mother Nature no other choice but to do it herself.

> "I have no doubt that it is a part of the destiny of the human race, in its gradual improvement, to leave off eating animals, as surely as the savage tribes have left off eating each other when they came in contact with the more civilized."
>
> —Henry David Thoreau, *Walden*

PART III

Taking Action: What Can We Do?

8

WHY DID NO ONE TELL
YOU THIS BEFORE?

"Everybody is ignorant, only on different subjects."

—Will Rogers

Where do we learn what to eat? More than likely, you first heard about what's good for you from your mother. As you grew older, you probably learned new information from your schoolteacher, your friends, and your family doctor. Because you trusted them, you expected to hear only the truth. In return, they believed what they were saying was best for you. As you became an adult, you heard information that reinforced these beliefs from other sources like your college professors, your new doctor, and your favorite anchor on the evening news. So why haven't any of the people you trust told you the facts about nutrition and the many interrelated global problems covered in this book? The answer is complicated in some ways but pretty simple in others. In a single word, it all begins with *money*.

From earliest childhood you have been inundated with ads promoting the health benefits of certain foods, ads from drug companies for pills to treat a wide assortment of ailments, and news stories that contain a never-ending flow of contradictory information about the effects of certain foods in your diet. But you probably have heard very little about the health-promoting power of a whole-foods, plant-based diet. Why is that?

Sadly, the people you trust were only telling you what they had been taught. This is not a story of conspiracy or of suspected misconduct on the part of any individual, company, institution, or branch of the government. This is a story of confusion that develops when an enormously complicated and interconnected group of organizations in a free market environment has zero financial incentive to promote the highest possible level of health.

Dr. T. Colin Campbell sums up the situation that exists today in the United States and, to an extent, in other Western countries:

> The entire system—government, science, medicine, industry and media—promotes profits over health, technology over food and confusion over clarity. Most, but not all, of the confusion about nutrition is created in legal, fully disclosed ways and is disseminated by unsuspecting, well-intentioned people, whether they are researchers, politicians or journalists. The most damaging aspect of the system is not sensational, nor is it likely to create much of a stir upon its discovery. It is a silent enemy that few people see and understand.[238]

While no organization within that "entire system" has a financial incentive to make you healthy, virtually all of them have an incentive to make the overall system bigger—by producing greater sales, earning bigger profits, and creating more jobs. Without a doubt, every doctor wishes to see every one of his or her patients cured of their disease and healthy. Unfortunately, our system doesn't provide the doctor with the tools needed to make that happen.

After spending many years and a small fortune on their education, those well-intentioned doctors work in a system whereby they earn a living by doing what they have been taught—diagnosing problems, writing prescriptions, and conducting procedures. Teaching patients how to take charge of their own health was never a part of their curriculum; nor would they be able to earn a living if they advocated it in their own practice. Please understand that this chapter is not about blaming doctors. Rather, it takes a hard look at a system that evolved over the past century. Understanding how this system emerged will help you develop the conviction you will need to successfully chart your own course.

Health by the Numbers

Dr. Campbell devotes the entire last third of *The China Study* to the question "Why haven't you heard this before?"[239] Why is the answer to this question so important? Because it determines what you will do with everything you have read so far, and it affects what course you will take in the future. A good place to start is to address the cost of health-care and the incredibly complex system that has developed to help us live longer.

Arguably, the cost of health-care is the number-one problem in the United States. *Forbes* noted in July 2009, "When asked about the federal government's long-term budget problem, Barack Obama always responds that it is essentially a health issue. Unless we fix the health-care system, he says, we cannot get control of the budget."[240] The article sums up the issue as follows:

> Health-care reform would be relatively easy if we were starting from scratch. But we aren't. We not only have to design a new system if we hope to lower costs without impairing health-care quality, but we also have to figure out how to get from here to there given that we have an enormously complicated health system involving massive

government programs along with huge health insurance companies, increasing numbers of businesses dropping or reducing their health-care benefits to workers, and a large and growing population of people with no health insurance at all.[241]

This enormously complicated system is composed of far more than just doctors, nurses, and hospitals. The system also includes close interactions with the food industry, the pharmaceutical industry, and health insurance companies. A huge amount of money is at stake, and millions of jobs are on the line throughout this vast, interconnected system.

The numbers involved are staggering. In 2008, health-care provided 14.3 million jobs for wage and salary workers. Ten of the twenty fastest-growing occupations are health-care related. Health-care will generate another 3.2 million jobs by 2018.[242] All this adds up to a total cost of health-care in the United States of an estimated $2.7 trillion in 2010.

How about the food industry? According to Marion Nestle in *Food Politics*, the term refers to companies that produce, process, manufacture, sell, and serve foods, beverages, and dietary supplements. The term also encompasses the entire collection of enterprises involved in supporting all of the above (for example, companies that produce fertilizer for growing feed for the cows). Citing data from the USDA Economic Research Service, Nestle reports, "This vast 'food-and-fiber' system generates a trillion dollars or more in sales every year, accounts for 13% of the U.S. gross national product (GNP), and employs 17% of the country's labor force."[243] With 154 million people in the 2010 workforce, that computes to almost 19 million employees.

In addition to 33 million people working in health-care and the food industries, almost 1 million employees work in pharmaceutical and health insurance careers. According to 2008 Bureau of Labor Statistics data, the pharmaceutical industry accounts for almost 400,000 employees. The insurance industry has been growing like wildfire in recent years. According to an article on the website of the Economic Policy Institute, employment in health insurance grew 52 percent in the ten years from 1997 to 2007, reaching 444,000 in August 2007.[244]

The grand totals—for health-care, food, pharmaceutical, and health insurance industries—come to almost $4 trillion in revenue and close to 35 million jobs. That's roughly 25 percent of the nation's GDP and one out of every five jobs in the United States. With these incredibly large numbers in mind, it is sobering to realize that not a single one of those 35 million employees has a financial incentive to promote health and reduce disease. It is indeed a complicated web we have woven—a system designed to address symptoms rather than causes.

Playing the Percentages

What would happen to the medical industry if 70 to 80 percent of our health-care costs simply went away? That is the potential reduction in health-care costs estimated by Dr. Campbell in the recent movie *Forks over Knives* if everyone in the United States adopted a whole-foods, plant-based diet. Suddenly, millions of health-care workers would be looking for jobs in other fields. What about the insurance companies? You might think that since they pay the claims, they would have an incentive to see that the procedures and medications cost as little as possible. Dr. John McDougall shed some light on that topic with a real-life example. In 1986, while working at the St. Helena Hospital in northern California, Dr. McDougall established an excellent track record of reversing chronic illnesses such as heart disease and type 2 diabetes. His program consisted solely of a shift to a plant-based diet. After comparing the cost of his highly successful program to the conventional treatment paradigm, he concluded that the insurance companies involved would greatly prefer a $5,000 expense that cured the disease to a $45,000 bypass that would only provide temporary relief.

So he began talking with insurance company representatives about adding his noninvasive program to the list of programs that would be covered by the patients' medical insurance. After preparing reams of information, analyses, and presentation materials highlighting the dramatic superiority of his program over the much costlier surgical treatments, he was naturally expecting a favorable response.

He was stunned when he received the first reply from a claims manager: "We're not interested; this is not the kind of program we can include in our coverage." When he asked the representative why not, he replied, "In order to stop the chest pains by your methods, you have to get the patients' cooperation; patients must change their diets, and I don't believe they will. For the bypass surgeon to stop the chest pains, all he has to do is get the patient to lie down on the operating room table. No willpower necessary." Not giving up easily, Dr. McDougall said, "But there are some patients who would much rather eat oatmeal, minestrone soup, and bean burritos and go for a daily walk than expose the inside of their chest to stale operating room air and risk death and brain damage. Don't you think they should be given an option, especially with the savings for your company?" After they went back and forth for a bit, the insurance representative made his position perfectly clear: "You don't get it, McDougall; you don't understand the business. We take a piece of the pie, and the bigger the pie, the more we get."[245]

We take a piece of the pie, and the bigger the pie, the more we get. That sentence speaks volumes about what is wrong with our extended health-care system; the future livelihood of everyone involved depends on that "pie" continuing to get bigger. The crux of the problem is that the health-care system does not provide incentives for improving the health of the patient. The only incentive for every segment of the extended system is to generate more revenue. That means more procedures, more drugs, and more hospital stays. That also explains why the health insurance business is booming these days. Insurance companies are making money hand over fist while American patients are shelling out a greater percentage of their checks for health-care than has any other culture of people in the history of the world.

The insurance companies are not the right guardians to lower the overall cost of health-care. Consider the automobile insurance business. If electronically controlled automobiles (with zero possibility of accidents) were to replace all of the cars in the world, what would happen to the auto insurance business? It would shrink to a mere shadow of its former self. The same would happen to the health insurance industry if everyone became healthy. If everyone were healthy, the risks would be lowered, and insurance companies couldn't justify their rates.

The enormous complexity of the system includes another key player. We all have seen the ubiquitous ads on television urging, "Ask your doctor if this drug is right for you." If ever a business was built on addressing symptoms rather than causes, it is the pharmaceutical industry.

Beware the Messenger

Doctors make up one of the most highly respected groups of professionals in the country, and they should be. Most of them enter the medical field to help people, and they spend many years and lots of money educating themselves for a satisfying career in their chosen field. Now they find themselves in a system that seems to encourage making money more than it does promoting health. The system rewards writing prescriptions, both giving their patients what they want—a palliative to what ails them—and putting more money in their own pocket.

After summarizing the wealth of published research that suggests that most of our chronic diseases are a result of poor nutrition, not poor genes or bad luck, Dr. Campbell asks, "So why doesn't the medical system take nutrition seriously? Four words: money, power, ego and control. While it is unfair to generalize about individual doctors, it is safe to say that the system they work in, the system that currently takes responsibility for promoting the health of Americans, is failing us."[246]

Part of that failure has to do with the cozy relationship that has developed between mainstream medicine and the drug industry in the past forty years. Dr. McDougall is quoted frankly on that topic in *The China Study*: "The problem with doctors starts with our education. The whole system is paid for by the drug industry, from education to research. The drug industry has bought the minds of the medical profession. It starts the day you enter medical school. All the way through medical school everything is supported by the drug industry."[247]

A 2009 article in the *New York Times* reports on an example at Harvard. "In a first-year pharmacology class at Harvard Medical School, Matt Zerden grew wary as the professor promoted the benefits of cholesterol drugs and seemed to belittle a student who asked about side effects . . . Mr. Zerden's minor stir four years ago has lately grown into a full-blown movement by more than 200 Harvard Medical School students and sympathetic faculty, intent on exposing and curtailing the industry influence in their classrooms and laboratories."[248]

The practice of taking money from the drug industry is widespread at Harvard and other prominent medical schools. "[N]o one disputes that many individual Harvard Medical faculty members receive tens or even hundreds of thousands of dollars a year through industry consulting and speaking fees. Under the school's disclosure rules, about 1,600 of 8,900 professors and lecturers have reported to the dean that they or a family member had a financial interest in a business related to their teaching, research or clinical care. The reports show 149 with financial ties to Pfizer and 130 with Merck."[249]

Noted heart specialist Dr. Dean Ornish shows how the pharmaceutical industry influences far more than just education. "Drug companies are the major advertisers in all medical journals. They fund clinical trials to determine the effectiveness of their drugs and they pay these researchers to speak at hospitals and medical schools. And if a drug company that makes a cholesterol-lowering drug provides most of the funds to conduct research on the effectiveness of that drug, then there is a potential for bias, even if unwittingly, despite independent monitoring committees that sometimes oversee these studies."[250]

Dr. John Abramson, clinical instructor at Harvard Medical School, explains in his book, *Overdo$ed America: The Broken Promise of American Medicine*, "When corporate partners fund the flow of information, the message is likely to accentuate treatment strategies that are in their interest and downplay those that are not."[251]

Marcia Angell, a Harvard faculty member and former editor in chief of the *New England Journal of Medicine*, gives an example of how this plays out in the real world in her book *The Truth about the Drug Companies*. She cites a large National Institutes of Health (NIH) trial of ways to prevent type 2 diabetes. Three groups were used. Two got drugs, and the other did not. Of the two that received drugs, one of them did slightly better than the other. But what about the group that didn't get drugs? She reports, "[T]he third group did much better than either of the other two. They were placed on a moderate diet and exercise program . . . In other words, diet and exercise were better than the drug. But trying diet and exercise instead of a drug is not likely to happen in real life. Drenched as we all are in prescription drug promotions, both doctors and patients are far more likely to go for the [drug]. Besides, insurers don't usually pay for diet and exercise programs."[252]

That last sentence sums up why no one in the system advocates diet and lifestyle approaches to health-care, even though they have been proven to be effective. There is no money. Dr. Abramson tells how the healthy lifestyle approaches are handled in the field of heart disease:

The problem is that the current medical recommendations, public education campaigns, drug advertisements, and news of break-throughs in the prevention of heart disease give the benefits of a healthy lifestyle just enough lip service to preempt criticism that these issues are being ignored. The end result is that doctors and patients are being distracted from what the research really shows: physical fitness, smoking cessation, and a healthy diet trump nearly every medical intervention as the best way to keep coronary heart disease at bay.[253]

Dr. Angell places some of the blame for the "cozy relationship" between pharmaceutical companies and practitioners on the fact that doctors are under a lot of pressure in today's world of managed care and that the drug prescription method is perhaps the only workable option they have. "In my view, we have become an overmedicated society. Doctors have been taught only too well by the pharmaceutical industry, and what they have been taught is to reach for a prescription pad. Add to that the fact that most doctors are under great time pressure because of the demands of managed care, and they reach for that pad very quickly."[254]

Dr. Angell also directs part of the blame at the patients. They have been brainwashed by television commercials and feel that they deserve to get a prescription every time they want one. "Patients have also been well taught by the pharmaceutical industry's advertising," she says. "They have been taught that if they don't leave the doctor's office with a prescription, the doctor is not doing a good job. The result is that too many people end up taking drugs when there may be better ways to deal with their problems."[255]

The bottom line is that we have come a long way from the time of Hippocrates, who said, "Your food will be your medicine, and your medicine will be your food." Dr. Abramson sums up the mutual embrace of doctors and pharmaceutical companies with a quote from a 2003 article in the *British Medical Journal*: "Twisted together like the snake and the staff, doctors and drug companies have become entangled in a web of interactions as controversial as they are ubiquitous."[256]

A Tower of Babel

The idea of strange bedfellows also applies when we consider the interactions among the massive food industry, the United States Department of Agriculture (USDA), and the elite world of nutritional science. First, as Dr. Caldwell Esselstyn explains, scientists have made a number of attempts to bring nutritional recommendations more into line with what clinical trials have actually determined. However, "[i]n every case, intensive lobbying by industry—the producers and purveyors of dairy products, meat, and poultry—has caused those who set the standards to pull their punches. To put it quite simply, the fox is in the henhouse. Nowhere is this more apparent than at the United States Department of Agriculture."[257]

Since the late 1970s, the USDA has been issuing the official government guidelines on what U.S. citizens should be eating. So who is running the USDA? In a 2004 *Nutrition Action Healthletter*, a publication of the Center for Science in the Public Interest, Michael Jacobson revealed the names and backgrounds of the top executives at the USDA. Every one of the top officers had previously been employed by the dairy, meat, or poultry industry.[258] Dr. Esselstyn goes on to state his opinion on the matter: "The Department of Agriculture, which by definition is supposed to protect and promote the nation's agricultural interests, should disqualify itself from responsibility for setting nutrition standards."[259] He notes, "As long ago as 1991 . . . proposed changes in the food pyramid would have relegated meat and dairy foods to lesser importance. But by the time the lobbying was finished, the USDA agreed on a misleading compromise for the new proposals that still emphasized consumption of animal protein."[260]

Marion Nestle, professor of sociology and nutrition, food studies, and public health at NYU, has worked as a policy advisor to the Department of Health and Human Services and as a member of nutrition and science advisory committees to the USDA and the FDA. She explains how the system works to influence the consumer in *Food Politics*: "We select diets in a marketing environment in which billions of dollars are spent to convince us that nutrition advice is so confusing, and eating healthfully so impossibly difficult, that there is no point in bothering to eat less of one or another food product or category."[261]

How do academia and science fit into this picture? About ten years ago, Dr. Campbell heard that his for-credit course in plant-based nutrition, which had been extremely popular among Cornell students for seven years, had been suddenly canceled by the administration, who didn't even inform him of their decision to drop it. He learned the news from a student who was trying to sign up for the course. He immediately contacted the department head who had authorized the cancellation.

When Colin confronted the department head asking for the reason, he said nothing. But it was well known that he was a substantial consultant to the dairy industry and, simultaneously, chair of major food recommendation committees (e.g., Dietary Guidelines/Food Pyramid committee of the USDA and nutritional recommendations of the National Academy of Sciences). And he had made clear his defense of dairy-related companies in projects like Nestle and Kraft.

Throughout an illustrious career of almost a half century, Dr. Campbell has distinguished himself by producing over 400 scientific research papers. Because he is such an esteemed scientist, he has been very successful in obtaining funding from the nation's number-one source for all biomedical and nutrition-related research (responsible for 80 to 90 percent), the NIH. The NIH is composed of twenty-seven separate institutes and centers, including its two largest, the National Cancer Institute (NCI) and the National Heart, Lung and Blood Institute (NHLBI). Yet none of those institutes and centers at the NIH is devoted to nutrition. With a total budget of $28 billion in 2004, only 3.6 percent was slated for nutrition research, despite findings that demonstrate the pivotal nature of nutrition in health.

The influence that food companies have on nutritional researchers is similar to the sway that pharmaceutical companies have over clinical trials. Nutrition conferences rely on industry support from food companies, as Marion Nestle reveals. She explains: "Food, beverage, and supplement companies buy space at exhibits; place advertisements in program books; underwrite coffee breaks, meals, and receptions; sponsor research awards and student prizes; and provide bags, pens, and other meeting souvenirs—for which they are thanked in program books."[262] She describes one conference of the American Society for Nutritional Sciences, which offered research sessions sponsored by trade associations such as the National Dairy Council and the National Cattlemen's Beef Association. Nestle's 500–page book is filled with countless examples of the cozy relationships between those who produce our food and the nutritional scientists who conduct research and create reports that affect the sales potential of the food products involved.

The big question is how much does industry sponsorship influence research and opinions? Nestle answers, "This question demands careful consideration if for no other reason than sponsorship by industry is so common. A 1996 survey found that nearly 30% of university faculty members accept industry funding; another found 34% of the primary authors of 800 papers in molecular biology and medicine to be involved in patents, to serve on advisory committees, or to hold personal shares in companies that might benefit from the research."[263] The rubber meets the road when the industry sponsors use the research results to advertise their products. Nestle cites one full-page ad in the *New York Times* that boldly states, "A groundbreaking study in the *Journal of the American Medical Association* proves that using margarine instead of butter *significantly lowers cholesterol*. The debate is over . . . the results proved once and for all that soft margarine is clearly the healthier choice . . . everyone in your family can feel good about eating it." The sponsor was a trade group identified by its website, Margarine.org.[264]

The ties that bind the government to the food industry are also shown in the massive farm subsidies we all hear so much about. By providing incentives to the producers of primarily meat and dairy products, the government enables the U.S. consumer to better afford these products. According to the Physicians Committee for Responsible Medicine (PCRM), a nonprofit organization that encourages preventive medicine, conducts clinical research, and advocates higher ethics and competence standards in research, "Between 1995 and 2004, nearly three-quarters of Farm Bill agricultural subsidies for food went for feed crops and direct aid supporting meat and dairy production. Less than half of 1 percent subsidized fruit and vegetable production."[265] Using the Farm Bill subsidy numbers, the PCRM produced the image in Figure 8.1, which explains at least part of the reason salad calories cost more than hamburger calories. Our government is supporting the industries that produce the least healthy foods.

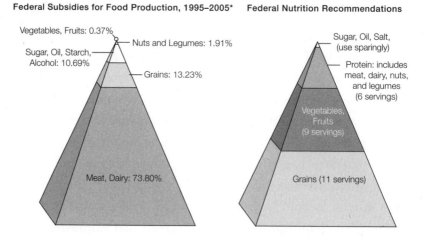

Figure 8.1 Why Does a Salad Cost More Than a Big Mac?[266]

The PCRM goes on to report: "The Farm Bill's skewed system of subsidies helps explain why unhealthy foods are often cheap and plentiful, while healthy foods are more expensive and less available. The priorities in the subsidy system stand in stark contrast to the federal government's own advice on nutrition."[267] As with dietary guidelines, there are a lot of politics and a lot of money involved. As Marion Nestle points out, "No matter who owns them, food companies lobby government and agencies, and they become financially enmeshed with experts on nutrition and health."[268]

A recent example of how well our government looks after our best interests was reported by the *New York Times* in late 2010. As the story goes, an organization by the name of Dairy Management was called in to help Domino's Pizza address its lagging sales. They worked with Domino's management on a program that added 40 percent more cheese to their pizzas and required a $12 million marketing campaign to promote it to the public. Apparently, the campaign worked; the article reports, "Consumers devoured the cheesier pizza, and sales soared by double digits. 'This partnership is clearly working,' Brandon Solano, the Domino's vice president for brand innovation, said in a statement to the *New York Times*."[269] But there's more to this story.

It turns out that Dairy Management is a part of the USDA. As the article explains:

Dairy Management, which has made cheese its cause, is not a private business consultant. It is a marketing creation of the United States Department of Agriculture—the same agency at the center of a federal anti-obesity drive that discourages over-consumption of some of the very foods Dairy Management is vigorously promoting ... The organization's activities, revealed through interviews and records, provide a stark example of inherent conflicts in the Agriculture Department's historical roles as both marketer of agriculture products and America's nutrition police.[270]

The article goes on to explain just how much cheese we're consuming: "Americans now eat an average of 33 pounds of cheese a year, nearly triple the 1970 rate. Cheese has become the largest source of saturated fat."[271] Clearly, our system is out of control, it continues to get worse, and our tax dollars are paying for it.

Dr. Campbell summarizes the problem: "Our institutions and information providers are failing us. Even cancer organizations, at both the national and local level, are reluctant to discuss or even believe this evidence. Food as a key to health represents a powerful challenge to conventional medicine, which is fundamentally built on drugs and surgery . . . The widespread communities of nutrition professionals, researchers and doctors are, as a whole, either unaware of this evidence or reluctant to share it. Because of these failings, Americans are being cheated out of information that could save their lives."[272]

In September 2010, a story broke in the news, somewhat by accident, about former president Bill Clinton and his recent decision to switch to a plant-based diet to provide his body with the ability to heal itself. He publicly acknowledged in interviews, including one on CNN, that he made this dietary change after reading the books written by Campbell, Esselstyn, and Ornish (one of his consulting physicians since 1993).[273] His decision is an example of an individual choice based on the facts and not on news influenced by lobbying. Our healthcare system needs to shift its focus away from generating revenue and place more emphasis on improving health. Rather than continuing to argue about who pays, the system should provide incentives based on improved health at the best possible value.

Instead of improving, our health continues to deteriorate—yet the costs keep going up. While the millions of individuals working within the health-care system would certainly like to see the health of everyone improve and the related costs go down, the overall system within which they work simply doesn't provide the incentives to make that happen. Further, no individual or organization within this vast complex has the power to change it in any significant way.

That leaves the consumer. Particularly in the wealthier nations of the OECD, most citizens have the freedom and the financial means to choose what they want to eat. And through the efforts of brave pioneers like Campbell, Esselstyn, Fuhrman, Ornish, McDougall, Barnard, and others, those citizens are learning truths about nutrition that they have never heard before. They are learning that they can take charge of their own health. With more and more people choosing health-promoting whole plants, eventually we will reach a tipping point.

Then the free market will respond and will deliver the goods that the citizens demand. This will set off a positive domino effect whereby people become healthier, the cost of health-care goes down, the damage to the environment is lessened, we consume fewer fossil fuels in the production of our food, we feed many more people on the same amount of land, and we end the suffering of animals in our factory farms. Now you know the facts about the world-changing power of the whole-foods, plant-based diet. And you have the power to help change the world with those facts.

Why haven't you heard all of this before? Given how nutritional and medical information on this crucial topic is generated and shared with the public in today's world, maybe the more accurate question would be: "How could you possibly expect to have heard this before?"

"A great deal of intelligence can be invested in ignorance."

—Saul Bellow

9

DECISION TIME

"Be the change you want to see in the world."

—Mahatma Gandhi

As you now know, the evidence supporting the shift to a whole-foods, plant-based diet is abundant and powerful. That leaves only the question of personal choice. Humans continue to consume, in ever-growing numbers, the toxic Western diet because they love the taste of cooked animal flesh, cheese, and other animal foods. Is that craving more important than promoting health, solving the health-care cost dilemma, nurturing our fragile environment, conserving our fossil fuels, reducing world hunger, and ending the horrible suffering of animals in our factory farms?

If you carefully consider all the factors, the answer is a resounding *no*. So how can you make a difference? Or perhaps the better question is how can such a large change be made? First, consider that the human craving for cooked flesh is just a habit. Bad habits, like chewing your fingernails, can be broken. The first step in eliminating a longtime habit is to make a firm decision to break it.

When deciding whether to give this improved diet a try, people often think of reasons for not changing. Some people are satisfied with their health and see no health reason to change. Some think switching to a plant-based diet would be an extreme change, and they are not sure if they are up to the challenge. Let's look at each of these concerns in turn.

I'm Healthy Already

You may be wondering why you need to change what you are eating. Maybe you are not overweight, have always tried to watch what you eat, and consider yourself to be in fairly good health. Even after reading about the many aspects of our health that are affected by what we eat, you're still not sure that this diet-style is right for you.

You should know that thin people, like everyone else, are not immune to the diseases caused by the rich Western diet. Skinny people have heart attacks and get cancer all the time; they also get diabetes, osteoporosis, and erectile dysfunction.

Then there's the phenomenon we call "vibrant health" that develops when one is eating a near-optimal diet. It's tough to explain what vibrant health feels like; everyone must experience it for himself or herself. Young people in their healthiest years don't spend a lot of time worrying about chronic disease or nursing homes, but many of them do make a decision to adopt a plant-based diet once they learn about the enormous impact food has on our world—beginning with their own health.

Tony Gonzalez, all-pro tight end, is an example of a young athlete who made the switch to a plant-based diet in the prime of a very successful career as a professional football player. Gonzalez is a veteran of ten Pro Bowls and is considered a future Hall of Famer. He changed his diet before the 2007 season after learning about *The China Study* from a fellow airline passenger. He read the book and then met with Dr. Campbell. In his book, *The All-Pro Diet*, he refers to Dr. Campbell as "an author who offered clear statistical and epidemiological evidence that my diet was a train wreck just waiting to happen."[274] He now eats an "almost vegan" diet—which earned him the nickname "China Study" from his teammates in Kansas City—and is stronger than ever. He lists the multiple benefits of his diet in his book. About endurance, he says, "You last longer while everyone else is getting tired." About focus, he says, "In the meeting room, in the classroom, at home, out on the field; wherever you are, you have greater ability to concentrate on what needs to be done." He also reports faster recovery time: "The day after working out hard or playing a tough game, you come back feeling fresh and full of energy. The other guys [are] hurting and moaning and, sure, you've got a few bumps and bruises, but you're ready to go again!"[275]

Is This Diet Too Extreme?

Bucking the norm is always tough, particularly when the norm involves an activity as popular as eating meat. People say, "I know I should eat better, but I could never go all the way to eating nothing but plants." When 95 percent or more of the population is consuming some variation of the typical Western diet, it takes a serious level of conviction to make a decision to shift to a completely plant-based diet. But is this diet too extreme or too weird? It is certainly not too extreme when you compare it to open-heart surgery, removal of a cancerous colon, the torture of 60 billion animals per year, or billions of starving human beings. Besides, this style of eating is not going to be considered extreme, or even unusual, for very much longer.

A good analogy is the fate of smoking in the past fifty years in the United States. Back in the 1950s, it seemed that almost all adults smoked cigarettes. It was considered the norm—even in the doctor's office, in the hospital, or right outside the church. It was permitted in all forms of public transportation, office workers smoked while on the job, and tough guys lit up in every motion picture of the day. At the time, it was weird *not* to smoke, but it's the opposite today. When people found out that smoking would kill them, they mysteriously didn't need a cigarette with their coffee any longer.

Studies show that every week approximately 19,000 Americans are adopting a plant-based diet. The number of vegetarians in the United States is growing at about 1 million per year—roughly a 14 percent growth rate. The movement has already gained a lot of momentum among eighteen- to twenty-four-year-old college students. As noted previously, approximately 18 percent of all college students in the nation consider themselves vegetarian. That's almost six times the national average of 3.2 percent. This rapidly growing trend among thoughtful young people is a harbinger of what lies ahead. Bill Clinton was the latest high-profile figure to publicly announce his conversion. A few days after the previously mentioned interview with CNN, Brian Williams remarked on *NBC Evening News*, "Notice that our former president is looking trimmer. He has lost twenty-four pounds, says that he is eating a plant-based, meatless, nondairy diet to keep his heart healthy." With a former president of the United States now on board, this trend could gain even more momentum. The question isn't if the day is coming; it's when you decide to take action to protect yourself.

Pesticides, Pollution, and Filth

That's fine for college kids, you might say, but you know of other factors that make you cautious. One major reason is the rightful concern about the cancer-promoting toxins and pesticides sprayed on the fruits and vegetables we consume. Although this is a problem, it pales in comparison to the toxins and pesticides found in animal foods. Dr. Fuhrman makes a good point: "If you are concerned about pesticides and chemicals, keep in mind that animal products, such as dairy and beef, contain the most toxic pesticide residues. Because cows and steers eat large amounts of tainted feed, certain pesticides and dangerous chemicals are found in higher concentrations in animal foods."[276]

John Robbins agrees:

At each successive stage up the food chain, the concentration of toxic chemicals is greatly increased. Thus, [a] fish will accumulate in its body the total amount of poisons accumulated by all the thousands of smaller fish it eats . . . Predator birds who eat fish often ingest extremely high concentrations of these deadly substances. By the same token, a cow or chicken or pig will retain in its flesh all the pesticides it has ever consumed or absorbed, and factory farm animals will build up especially high concentrations of chemical toxins for several reasons.[277]

Among those reasons, he lists the fact that they are fed great quantities of fish meal, and their other feeds are often grown on land heavily sprayed with the most dangerous pesticides.[278]

Dr. Fuhrman talks about the toxins in seafood: "Fish is one of the most polluted foods we eat, and it may place consumers at high risk for cancers. Scientists have linked tumors in fish directly to the pollutants ingested along the aquatic food chain, a finding confirmed by the National Marine Fisheries Service Laboratory."[279] Howard Lyman agrees: "The municipal wastes and agricultural chemicals that we flush into our waters become absorbed in the tissues of fish and shellfish and thus into most of the items on the menu at your favorite seafood restaurant. The *Consumer Reports* study found PCBs in 43 percent of salmon and 25 percent of swordfish. Catfish had significant levels of DDT, clams had high levels of lead, and 90 percent of swordfish contained mercury."[280]

We should also be concerned about fish for another reason. Have you ever wondered about that "fishy" smell in the supermarket? Why don't living fish smell that way when they are being pulled out of the water? That's because the fish in the supermarket have likely been dead for two weeks or more and are well along in the process of spoiling. Lyman cites a 1992 *Consumer Reports* study that found almost 40 percent of the fish samples from supermarkets were in the "beginning to spoil" range (when bacteria grows to 1 million colonies per gram). An additional 25 percent were even further along, with more than 27 million colonies per gram. In addition, nearly half the fish tested were contaminated by bacteria from human or animal feces.[281]

Yes, pesticides are a problem in both plant and animal foods, but the larger problem is by far in the latter. John Robbins sums it up: "Recent studies indicate that of all the toxic chemical residues in the American diet, almost all, 95% to 99%, comes from meat, fish, dairy products and eggs."[282] According to Julie Gerberding, director of the CDC, "Eleven of the last twelve emerging infectious diseases that we're aware of in the world, that have had human health consequences, have probably arisen from animal sources."[283] All this pollution and contamination add up to a very unhealthy situation that can be largely avoided with a shift to a plant-based diet.

Thinking of the Children

Among the most important reasons to adopt a plant-based diet is the effect it will have on your children and all your descendants that follow. Have you looked at a kids' menu lately? Virtually all of them are lacking in vital nutrients and often don't include a single healthy item to choose.

The kids' menus of today almost always contain the following six items, and oftentimes, nothing else: cheeseburger, french fries, cheese pizza, chicken nuggets, fried fish, and macaroni and cheese. The top two choices of beverage are milk and soda. When eating away from home, many kids rarely consume a single calorie from whole plant foods. This typical menu has become so ubiquitous that parents everywhere have accepted it as the normal food for children. This is not *normal* food at all; it's a recipe for disaster. Table 9.1 shows nutrition facts for these six foods. All six are heavy in fat as a percentage of total calories, all have saturated fat, and all but one contain cholesterol. If such foods were only an occasional "treat," such poor choices might be tolerable. Tragically, though, this is what the kids are eating all time—even at school. This is why the obesity and diabetes rates for children are soaring.

Table 9.1 Typical Kids' Menu Items[284]

Menu Item	Fat (%)	Saturated Fat (grams)	Cholesterol (mg)
Burger King cheeseburger	32	8	50
McDonald's french fries*	43	2	0
Cheese pizza	43	6	10
Chicken nuggets	53	3	34
Long John Silver's fish	51	4	30
KFC macaroni and cheese	40	3	10

A potato without the oil contains 1 percent fat.

Today's kids are not even eating as healthily as their parents do, averaging a smaller percentage of their calories from whole plants. And most of their plant-based calories come from french fries, in which 43 percent of the calories are from fat. They might occasionally eat a few baby carrots and celery sticks with ranch dressing, but one ounce of ranch dressing has ninety-four calories, and 88 percent of them come from fat. A child would need to eat at least twenty of those baby carrots with that one ounce of ranch dressing to reduce the percentage of calories from fat from that snack down to 50 percent.

If your children have been eating these kinds of foods for a long time, you must be willing to make a strong effort to shift them over to a health-promoting diet. And unless you enthusiastically adopt this healthful plant-based diet yourself, your kids won't see a reason to make many changes at all. The remedy to the deplorable state of our children's diets lies primarily with the level of concern of their parents.

You can teach your kids to take charge of their health at a very young age. You can show them how to avoid colds, run faster, think better, maintain a trim body, and avoid the ravages of heart disease and cancer down the road. In short, you can be the model your children want to follow.

Baby Steps or Rapid Change?

Okay, you've made up your mind and are wondering what to do next. What level of change do you think you can handle? And how quickly should you make that change? Some people make the shift almost immediately, and others take a more gradual approach. Although some have experienced success with the gradual approach, the experts quoted in this book all agree that taking baby steps is not the best way to go for a number of reasons.

Dr. McDougall puts it this way: "If you are sincere about making the change, do so with 100% of your effort. Many people feel that it would be easier for them to slide into this diet plan gradually. Unfortunately, we seldom manage to discard old ways and old established tastes unless 100% of our effort is devoted to the change and unless, from the beginning, we make a clear break from our old behavior."[285] He adds that a smoker who cuts down to four cigarettes a day only goes through slow torture and rarely quits completely.

Another point to consider is that if you don't give this diet a serious 100 percent trial, then you may never experience the many aspects of vibrant health that it can deliver. As Dr. Ornish says:

In our research, we learned that it is often easier for people to make comprehensive changes in diet and lifestyle than to make only moderate ones. At first, this may seem like a paradox, but it makes sense when you understand why. If you make only *moderate* changes in lifestyle—for example, reducing fat intake from the typical American diet of about 40 percent of calories as fat to the conventional dietary guidelines of 30 percent fat—then you have the worst of both worlds. You feel deprived and hungry because you are not eating everything you want and are used to, but you're not making changes big enough to feel that much better or to significantly affect your weight or how you feel (or, for that matter, your cholesterol, blood pressure, or heart disease).[286]

But Dr. Ornish also makes it clear in his latest book, *The Spectrum*, that it is not an "all or nothing" proposition. As he told me recently, "In all of our research studies, we learned that the more people changed their diet and lifestyle, the more they improved in objective measures . . . and the better they felt." He went on to say, "that what matters most is your overall way of eating and living—if you indulge yourself one day, eat healthier the next."

You'll also feel deprived if you choose to continue having your favorite animal foods a few times a week. As Dr. Campbell concludes, "[F]ollowing this diet requires a radical shift in your thinking about food. It's more work to just do it halfway. If you plan for animal-based products, you'll eat them—and you'll almost certainly eat more than you should . . . [Y]ou'll feel deprived. Instead of viewing your new food habit as being able to eat all the plant-based food you want, you'll be seeing it in terms of having to limit yourself, which is not conducive to staying on the diet long-term."[287]

Dr. Ornish agrees, advising that if you don't make the change completely, "you're clear about what you're giving up, but you aren't getting much positive reinforcement to make you feel like you're getting something back that's equal or better . . . In contrast, when you make *comprehensive* changes in diet and lifestyle . . . then you begin to feel so much better, so quickly, that the choices and benefits become much clearer."[288]

Finally, consider the following advice from William James, the father of American psychology: "[I]n the acquisition of a new habit, or the leaving off of an old one, we must take care to *launch ourselves with as strong and decided an initiative as possible.*" To this first step, he added a second: "Never suffer an exception to occur till the new habit is securely rooted in your life."[289]

You may be wondering how long it will take to get results from this improved diet. You will be delighted to know that some benefits will be noticeable right away, within a week or two. The experts quoted above recommend a serious commitment of anywhere from six weeks to four months, but again, they all recommend a completely plant-based diet during that period. The longer your trial period, the less likely you will return to your old, unhealthy way of eating. For best results, we recommend that you give it 100 percent of your effort for four months. Making the change rapidly at age fifty-eight, I found that I was still experiencing new benefits well beyond the six-week stage. The longer you have been on the toxic Western diet, the longer it may take to fully cleanse your system and start delivering the thrilling elements of vibrant health that you may have been missing for many years.

"Accept the challenges, so you may feel the exhilaration of victory."

—George S. Patton

10

LET'S DO IT!

"Always bear in mind that your own resolution to succeed
is more important than any other thing."

—Abraham Lincoln

Now that you know about the challenges and have chosen your
level of commitment, let's get started. This chapter provides
information, tips, and references aimed at helping you make
this new diet-style fun, easy, effective, and permanent. All the guidelines that follow were prepared based on the assumption that you will
give this new way of eating 100 percent of your effort for between six
weeks and four months.

As noted in Chapter 9, for best results, we recommended that you
make a four-month commitment. The longer the time, the more you
will notice the benefits—in many facets of your life. These benefits will
show you why you should make this new way of eating permanent. If
you've decided on a more gradual approach, this chapter will still be a
handy reference as you move forward.

Keeping It Simple

My friend Laura has been eating more plant-based foods because she wants to lose weight. For the past ten months, she has been gradually eliminating animal foods from her diet. She says she feels better, and friends tell her that she looks healthier. The problem is that she hasn't lost much weight. Recently, I asked her what she had eaten during the past twenty-four hours. The first two items she mentioned raised red flags. Her first calories of the day were derived from a granola breakfast bar, and her second meal consisted of a mixture of spinach, mushrooms, and eggs. According to the Nutrition Data website, the breakfast bar is 34 percent fat.[290] As for the other dish, the eggs constitute 80 percent of the meal's calories. And since eggs are 66 percent fat, over half the calories in the meal came from fat.[291] No one can expect to promote health or reduce weight with numbers like those.

Laura, like many vegetarians, is more concerned about what she is *not* eating (animal flesh in particular) and hasn't focused on maximizing her calories from highly nutritious, whole, plant-based foods. I gave her two very simple guidelines—two words and one number: whole plants and 20 percent. More specifically:

1. Eat lots of whole plants—in nature's package. Plan every meal around these health-promoting foods. Shoot for more than 80 percent of all calories in every meal from whole plants.
2. Keep fat calories below 20 percent of your total calories consumed. Dr. Esselstyn likes for his heart patients to achieve 10 percent; the average consumer of the Western diet comes closer to 40 percent. We have found 20 percent to be a reasonable number and not too difficult to achieve.

As I explained to Laura, you don't need to count calories all the time to figure out how you're doing. I told her to just analyze several of her favorite meals using the Nutrition Data website (NutritionData.com), learn how to adjust those meals to increase the whole-plant calorie percentage, and let nature take its course. For my typical breakfast and lunch meals, the percentage of calories from whole plant foods is about 95 percent, and the percentage of calories from fat is just over 9 percent. And that includes a little bit of very high-fat avocado and olives in my lunch almost every day.

If you hit 80 percent of calories or more from whole plant foods, you will be getting ten times more whole plant calories than the average consumer of the typical Western diet. You'll also be consuming well over fifty grams of colon-cleansing fiber and will probably never have constipation or heartburn again. I haven't even had the hiccups since I began eating this way.

Celebration—Not Deprivation

That's right, celebration. By choosing whole plants for the majority of your calories, you can eat all you want at every meal. If you're eating the right foods, it's almost impossible to eat too much. You don't have to count calories or ever feel like you're depriving yourself. When you're eating the right foods, your body will tell you when it's ready for more food.

You're on the threshold of a whole new way of thinking about what you eat and why you eat it. We have all grown up during an era of choosing food based on a single criterion—the pleasure of eating. Not surprisingly, food marketers have loaded up almost all of our foods with white flour, sugar, fat, and salt, which have resulted in unnatural cravings. But you can now intelligently choose what you eat.

The time has arrived for a new era of eating for the right reasons without sacrificing the many pleasures of dining that we all have grown to love. We should focus on promoting health by maximizing the consumption of the healthiest foods, and we have created a scoring system to help others understand this concept and turn over a *new leaf* in their lives. It is called the *4-Leaf Health Promotion Program*. Table 10.1 illustrates this simple concept, which will help you maximize the percentage of whole plant food calories in your diet while keeping your fat calories under control.

Table 10.1 The 4-Leaf Health Promotion Program

Diet Level	Calories from Whole Plants	What Results Can You Expect?[292]
4Leaf	80% or more	Representing a small minority of the population, people in this category tend to have trim bodies, enjoy vibrant health, have lots of energy, take no medications, are almost never sick, and will very likely live a long and healthy life.
3Leaf	60% to 79%	People in this group derive well over half of their calories from health-promoting, whole, plant-based foods and have experienced many benefits of a healthy diet. They are well on their way to the four-leaf level.
2Leaf	40% to 59%	Although probably making a serious effort to eat a healthy, balanced diet, people in this group are falling short of ensuring long-term vibrant health. With a little help, they probably will move quickly up the scale.
1Leaf	20% to 39%	Although eating better than most, people in this category consume nowhere near enough whole plant foods to provide much protection against disease, and they will need help to add more leaves.
No-Leaf	Zero to 19%	People in this group consume the typical Western diet, with meat and dairy at almost every meal. This destructive diet provides almost no fiber from whole plant foods and offers zero protection against chronic disease.

4Leaf The Foundation of the 4-Leaf Program

In Chapter 1, we told you the story of five trailblazing medical doctors who all discovered—after medical school—the power of plant-based nutrition to promote vibrant health and even reverse chronic disease. While some of these outstanding physicians may disagree on one or two minor aspects of plant-based nutrition, there is a vast amount of "common ground" on which they are all in total agreement. We have built our 4-leaf Program on that *common ground*.

After studying all of the published works of these great doctors, I have concluded that they all agree on this statement by Dr. T. Colin Campbell, "The closer we get to a diet of whole, plant-based foods the better off we will be." Hence our trademarked 4-leaf Program encourages our readers and clients to maximize the percent of their calories from these nutritious foods—simple, practical, flexible, and powerful.

As Dr. Joel Fuhrman has said many times, "You must get the majority of calories from unrefined plant food for optimal health." He adds, "Following a strict vegetarian diet is not as important as eating a diet rich in fresh fruits and vegetables." So that's the positive advice we want to build on in this program—focusing purely on maximizing the percent of your calories from the healthiest foods—and not placing your primary emphasis on the foods that you are avoiding. For more helpful information, tips, and tools, please visit our 4-leaf website at www.4leafprogram.com.

Here's how the 4-leaf Program works. If 80 percent or more of your calories are derived from whole plants, and less than 20% of your calories are derived from fat, you are eating at the 4-leaf level, which is the goal. We have been told our entire lives that we should eat more fruits and vegetables. We want to build on that simple, positive advice. Too often, people try to improve their diet by cutting out certain foods one at a time. They put a lot of thought into what they're avoiding but not nearly enough thought into what they should be maximizing—*whole plants*. Instead, think of each calorie as a fleeting opportunity to do something great for your body, giving it the health-promoting power of whole plants to nurture your 100 trillion cells.

Among other things; nurturing also means helping with the cell-replacement process. After learning that our bodies replace about 10 trillion of our cells every year, and knowing that we are what we eat, I wanted to find out how many cells are affected by each bite of food we take. So I counted my bites for a few days, did the math and came up with a staggering number. Roughly, the future health of 100 million cells is riding on every single bite you put into your mouth. So we want to help you make every bite count.

With this concept in mind, go to the Nutrition Data website (nutritiondata.com), and analyze a few of your typical meals. If you're eating the typical Western diet, it won't take you very long to add up the calories from the whole plants; and you will more than likely find that you are either at the no-leaf or 1-leaf level in our 4-leaf scoring system.

While adding up your calories from whole plants, calculate the percentage of your calories from fat for each meal, including the not-so-healthy animal-based foods and the highly processed plant-based foods. Just divide the calories from fat by the total calories shown on the nutrition facts panel for each food. The number you want (for a daily average) is 20 percent or less—far below that of the typical Western diet, which delivers 35 to 40 percent of its calories from fat. Shown below is a sample of the Nutrition Facts Panel that must appear on all packaged foods in the United States. Following that panel are two examples of food analyses—one healthy, the other not so healthy.

Sample Nutrition Facts Panel
Visit NutritionData.com to see the actual
panels of the two foods in our examples.

Nutrition Facts

Serving Size 125g

Amount Per Serving

Calories 65	Calories from Fat 2

	% Daily Value*
Total Fat 0g	0%
Saturated Fat 0g	0%
Trans Fat	
Cholesterol 0mg	0%
Sodium 1mg	0%
Total Carbohydrate 17g	6%
Dietary Fiber 3g	12%
Sugars 13g	
Protein 0g	

Vitamin A	1%	•	Vitamin C	10%
Calcium	1%	•	Iron	1%

*Percent Daily Values are based on a 2,000 calorie diet.
Your daily values may be higher or lower depending
on your calorie needs.

NutritionData.com

Food Analysis Examples

We chose one of the healthier items at Burger King for the first example: the original Whopper with no cheese. It even has a fair amount of whole plants, including tomatoes, lettuce, onions, sesame seeds, and pickles. For the second food scoring example, we use a banana.

As you can see, this is not rocket science. It's a simple matter of maximizing the percentage of your calories from whole plants. Using the Nutrition Data website, you can probably determine your 4-leaf score pretty quickly. If you have an idea how many calories you typically

Burger King Whopper, No Cheese
Calories from fat = 336
Total calories = 678

Percentage of calories from fat = 336 ÷ 678 = 50%
Calories from whole plants (tomato, lettuce, onion, seeds, pickles) = 14

Percentage of calories from whole plants = 14 ÷ 678 = 2%
The Whopper also contains 12 grams of saturated fat, 87 milligrams of cholesterol, 911 milligrams of sodium, and 12 grams of added sugars. These data put
it at the *no-leaf* level in our system.

Fresh Banana (Medium)
Calories from fat = 3
Total calories = 105

Percentage of calories from fat = 3 ÷ 105 = 3%
Calories from whole plants = 105

Percentage of calories from whole plants = 105 ÷ 105 = 100%
Bananas also contain zero saturated fat, zero cholesterol, 1 milligram sodium,
and 3 grams of dietary fiber. These numbers put bananas at the *4-leaf* without
a doubt.

consume per day, just add up the whole-plant calories from your meals
(breakfast, lunch, dinner, and snack) and divide by your total daily calories. Your analysis may look something like the one on the next page.

If you usually eat a sausage biscuit for breakfast, and your daily
snack is cheese and crackers, you won't need the Nutrition Data site or
a calculator to compute your whole-plant calories from those meals—
it will be zero in both cases. And the fat in those meals will likely make
up well over 50 percent of the calories.

ANALYSIS OF CURRENT DIET

Estimated daily calories = 2,500
Calories from whole plants
- Typical breakfast = 50
- Typical lunch = 75
- Typical dinner = 150
- Typical snack = 25

Total calories from whole plants = 300
Percentage of calories from whole plants = 300 ÷ 2,500 = 12%
Score on the *4-Leaf Program* scale = No Leaf

If your score is in the no-leaf range, please do not despair. You are not alone; in fact, you are in the large majority. But since you are in charge of what you eat, you can easily improve your score—and your health—by creating some healthier typical meals. When designing those meals, remember that we're talking about maximizing the percent of your calories from whole plant foods. First let's define what we mean by whole plant foods. Quite simply, our definition is *plant food ... still in nature's package.* So that includes all fresh fruit, greens, legumes, vegetables, nuts, seeds, and whole grains.

So what about plant-based foods like bread, pasta, and tofu? While not harmful like meat and dairy, these foods have been processed and simply don't contain the nutrient density and health-promoting qualities of those foods that are still in nature's package. Further, we have observed that many people who load up on these kinds of foods often-times don't get the results that they were expecting. Do include in your meals whole-grain brown rice or whole legumes such as black beans and all types of lentils, peas, and the like. Also load up on the green leafy vegetables and legumes. Lots of beans and greens are highly recommended.

Designing Some 3-Leaf and 4-Leaf Meals

There are lots of great 4-leaf recipes and meal-planning ideas in the books listed near the end of this chapter. But don't be afraid to design your own meals as well. When I began analyzing my meals a few years ago, I found the "My Recipe" function on Nutrition Data's website (nutritiondata.com) to be very helpful. This feature enables you to look at an entire meal as a single recipe. You create the recipe by adding in all the ingredients one at a time. Then you can look at the nutrition facts panel for the meal and easily calculate your percentage of calories from fat and your percentage of calories from whole plants. If you're consistently eating meals at the 3-leaf or 4-leaf level, you will be making your body very happy.

We've said that we don't consider this program to be vegetarian or vegan; rather, it's all about maximizing the percentage of your calories from whole plants. However, you will find that if you continue to make animal foods part of your normal routine, you will have a difficult time reaching the targets of 80 percent of calories from whole plants and less than 20 percent of calories from fat.

Dr. John McDougall makes a sensible point: "[W]hen I recommend a mostly vegetarian diet, I'm not asking people to do something bizarre, or out of the ordinary. All I'm asking is that we go back to doing what people have been doing for a million years or so. From the standpoint of long human experience, the American diet is the anomaly. It is the first time large numbers of humans have consumed so much animal foods, fat, refined foods, and artificial ingredients. The American diet is just a fad, soon to pass."[293]

Once again, our thinking behind the 4-leaf Program was to create something that was positive, simple, and easy to use. You will find that once you get into a healthy-eating routine, there is no need to do any daily tracking of calories. Just analyze a few of your new meals from time to time, and make sure they're at least at the 3-leaf level. One final thought: when you're eating at the 4-leaf level, you can simply eat all you want—when you want. And your body will reward you for the rest of your life. For more information on this program, please visit our website at www.4leafprogram.com.

Where to Start

Start out by evaluating your daily and weekly eating routine—what, where, when, with whom, and how much? You need to go through this process for each meal of the day as well as for snacks. As you analyze the nutritional content of what you're eating, you'll be surprised by where all your calories have been coming from. Take, for example, that salad you've been eating for lunch. Most salads available in restaurants are loaded with unhealthy, fat-laden items like cheese, eggs, meat, and oily dressing. But you might be surprised at the source of calories in even a healthy-looking salad.

The following is an analysis of a salad made up of a huge bowl of raw spinach, two whole plum tomatoes, a full cup of diced mushrooms, a half-cup of sliced cucumber, and one medium sliced carrot. It is topped off with a single ounce of French dressing.

- The salad has 269 total calories.
- 177 of those calories—66 percent of the total meal—come from the dressing.
- Only 92 of those calories come from the veggies.
- 98 percent of the calories in the dressing are from fat.

So two-thirds of the calories from the salad are from the fat in the single ounce of salad dressing. How about the percentage of calories from whole plants? Sadly, this huge salad derives only 34 percent of its energy from whole plants. Granted, that's higher than the average of 5 percent for most consumers of the typical Western diet, but it's nowhere near your target of 80 percent or more.

Again, you don't need to count portions or calories and keep track of any kind of data once you've established this powerful diet as a routine part of your life. Once you analyze a few meals, you learn pretty quickly what you need to do to hit your target. After you've worked out your routine, you can simply eat all you want of your favorite kinds of health-promoting foods.

According to several online calorie-needs calculators, I need 2,550 calories a day. In the previous salad example, had we chosen lime juice or some kind of vinegar for the dressing, the entire salad would have contained only 100 calories—certainly not enough to be considered a meal for someone who needs 2,550 calories from all meals combined. So you need to think about these factors in advance. Then you won't wonder why you're starving one hour after having a huge salad for lunch. To add more calories, you can add more calorie-rich whole-plant items to that salad—such as beans, whole-grain rice, grilled zucchini, eggplant, mushrooms, artichokes, potato, avocado, nuts, seeds, or olives. (Go easy on the last four, as they average 75 percent of their calories from fat.)

As you begin your new diet-style, record your baseline data as well—your weight and measurements, cholesterol levels, and blood pressure. All are almost certain to improve during your trial period and will continue to improve as you make these health-promoting habits a permanent part of your life. People often report their doctor's reaction to their improved biomarkers as "I don't know what you're doing, but whatever it is, keep doing it." You might also take some "before" pictures—and start putting money in your budget for buying some new clothes in a few months.

Meal Planning

What will you be eating? When and where will you eat it? You'll need to think through your daily routine for the week. Most people have a fairly set routine for the weekdays and a more flexible one for the weekends. My work as a writer and management consultant affords me a great amount of flexibility in terms of when and where I eat. On the other hand, my thirty-seven-year-old son, who eats almost exactly the way I do, works for a large public company in Boston and commutes to his office five days a week. Fortunately, they have a great in-house cafeteria, and he has plenty of healthy choices for lunch. My twenty-seven-year-old nephew, who travels the world out of New York for a prominent international consulting firm, is also a seasoned healthy eater and has no trouble finding the right kind of food.

After eating this way for almost eight years, I have established the following routine for the two meals that I eat at home every day. (I used the "My Recipe" function on the Nutrition Data website to compute the aggregate analysis for each meal.)

Breakfast. The morning starts with a large bowl of fresh, seasonal fruit at seven or eight. This meal delivers about 275 calories, 100 percent of which are whole plants, in nature's package. I prepare my second breakfast meal when I get hungry, which usually occurs around ten or eleven. That meal consists of a bowl of whole-grain oatmeal with a 50-50 mixture of water and unsweetened soy or almond milk. While visiting Dr. and Mrs. Esselstyn's family farm for breakfast one summer morning, I learned to enjoy those whole oats without cooking them. They're quite refreshing after soaking for a few minutes in the cold water and soy milk mixture. I load up that bowl with an assortment of raisins, berries, apples, or bananas (whatever's fresh), along with a sprinkle of ground flaxseed, from which I get my daily dose of omega-3s. On a typical day, my grand total food consumption prior to noon equals about 750 calories, almost all from whole plants.

Lunch. When you're consuming only health-promoting foods, you will find that even after eating all you want at every meal, your body will likely be ready for more food within three to four hours. Cued by that hunger signal from my body, my midday meal occurs between one thirty and three in the afternoon. It typically consists of a medley of steamed vegetables; whole-grain brown or wild rice; some variety of legume (beans); a few slices of eggplant; and a whole-wheat pita stuffed with raw or very slightly cooked spinach, along with a raw tomato, cucumber, and carrot and a very small amount of olive and avocado. This very enjoyable and satisfying meal delivers about 600 calories, bringing my halftime score to a very strong 4-leaf level.

HALFTIME (MIDDAY) SCORE

- Total calories consumed = 1,350
- Percentage of calories from whole plant foods = 95%
- Percentage of calories from fat = 9.4%
- Total grams of fiber = 55

Dinner. My meal planning factors in dining out in the evening at least five times a week. The restaurants I frequent understand my dietary preferences and do a phenomenal job of making me happy. Since what they serve me is not listed on the menu, invariably people sitting next to me at the bar will say, "I'll have what he's having." Tips on teaching your favorite restaurants to take good care of you will follow later in this chapter. But, for now, here is an example of how I have ordered a 4-leaf meal. Years ago, I noticed an attractive dish on our yacht club menu called Tiger Shrimp, served with grains, seaweed, and a medley of vegetables. I simply told the waiter that I would have the Tiger Shrimp, hold the shrimp, double up on the grains, vegetables, and seaweed and just have the chef adjust the price accordingly. After years of eating this way at my club, they now have the following entree on the printed menu, priced at $15, well below ALL the other entrees:

The Hicks Special
A selection of whole grains & fresh vegetables

What is my point in describing my own meal planning? It is to show how I can easily get the 2,550 calories that I need, with over 80 percent of them from whole plant foods. This routine delivers over 75 grams of fiber per day, with far less than 20 percent of the calories coming from fat. And if I can do it, so can you. As you go about doing your own meal planning, all seven books at the end of this chapter are good sources to explore. In addition to lots of recipes, they each provide useful meal-planning information.

Grocery Shopping

Always remember: if it goes into your shopping cart, it is almost certain to end up in your stomach. How you shop for food is very important, because once it's in your house, you will eat it. For that reason, one of the first steps in turning over a new leaf is getting rid of all the unhealthy items in your cupboards and your fridge. To avoid being wasteful, donate these foods to your favorite charity, or give them to a friend or family member. Don't just put them out of sight, though. Storing them in your basement, for instance, might be a subliminal message to your brain that this trial is only going to be temporary.

The next step is to sit down with a few recipe books and begin planning what you might like to prepare. Talk to people who are already eating this way, and ask them for ideas. Then, before formally beginning your challenge period, prepare a few samples of one or more of the new meals that you might like to have for breakfast, lunch, dinner, and snacks.

Now, armed with your plan of action, you are ready to head off to the grocery store. For your first trip, you're going to be thinking about two categories of food, and you should make a separate list for each:

1. The basics such as whole grains, dry beans, seasonings, salad dressings, and so on that you keep in your cupboard to prepare your meals on a daily basis. This list should not include any oils, sugar, salt, or any product containing dairy, white flour, or added sugar of any kind.
2. The fresh food that you plan to eat at home during the next week.

A word of caution: even in the best of supermarkets like Whole Foods and Trader Joe's, you will encounter thousands of attractively packaged foods that are simply not healthy for you. But in their defense, any large grocery chain would go out of business if it didn't supply all of its customers with exactly what they wanted. And for most, that still means meat, dairy, and highly processed foods at every meal. In most grocery stores, an estimated 90 percent of the calories being sold come from those unhealthy kinds of foods. You will need to be able to sort through those items to find the wonderful health-promoting foods for you and your family. First, a couple of general guidelines:

- Spend most of your time in the fresh produce section, selecting items that have no labels.
- When shopping in other areas of the store, look for the word "whole" in the ingredient list, and avoid purchasing items that have more than two or three ingredients. Most packaged breads today, for instance, have over twenty ingredients.

Fat in Whole Plants

Food Item	Calories from Fat (%)
Avocado	76
Almonds	72
Olives	70
Celery	11
Broccoli	10
Tomato	9
Carrots	3
Banana	3
Apple	3
Orange	3
Pear	2

Unlike animal-based foods, all of the above contain lots of healthy fiber and phytonutrients. They all contain protein too.

As you can see, the first three items are heavy in fat; you'll want to limit your consumption of these to keep your fat intake around the 15 percent target.

Source: NutritionData.com (details may vary based on brand chosen and type of preparation).

Learn how to properly read labels. Jeff Novick, a former manager at Kraft Foods with a long list of nutritional degrees and credentials, makes very good points about how to do this effectively. To start, don't believe anything on the front of the package. It includes words and phrases to make you think that you are buying a healthy product. The front of the package has everything to do with marketing and almost nothing to do with nutrition. Check the nutrition facts panel and the list of ingredients, which by law must be included on every package. Here is where you can find information to help you make the best choices about packaged food. Forget what the package says about the percentage of fat or that it says "fat free," and do a little math on your own. As noted previously, the nutrition facts panel contains total calories per serving and the number of calories from fat. Simply divide the fat calories by the total calories to get the percentage. You want to average less than 20 percent of your calories from fat. If you buy many items with 25 percent of calories from fat or more, you'll have a hard time hitting your goal.

An example of the tricks the food industry plays is in how 2 percent milk is labeled. When you do the math, you realize that 37.5 percent of the calories are from fat. The dairy folks compute the percentage of fat based on weight, leading you to believe that only 2 percent of the calories come from fat. Novick also warns you to watch out for the "PAM scam." The FDA allows any food with less than half a gram of fat per serving to put a zero in the nutrition box under calories per serving. Of course, the makers of cooking spray then take the liberty of calling this product "fat free" since their recommended serving size is a fourth of a second spray that delivers less than half a gram. Even though the five-ounce container delivers a total of 462 calories, amazingly, each serving contains 0 calories. To be fair, using cooking spray is a better choice than cooking everything in oil.[294]

One additive the food industry especially likes is sugar. As Michael Pollan explains in his book *In Defense of Food*, "[M]ore than half the sweeteners you consume come from corn."[295] He adds that most of the corn crop in the United States is used to feed livestock, and much of the rest goes into processed foods. Added sugars like corn fructose have become ubiquitous in virtually all categories of processed foods, particularly dry cereals, bread, nut milks like soy and almond, frozen dinners, and energy bars. It is almost impossible to find a breakfast cereal that doesn't contain at least seven grams of added sugar per serving. Looking at the Nutrition Data website, you find that healthy-sounding cereals such as Banana Nut Crunch and Raisin Bran contain twelve and seventeen grams of sugar respectively.[296] The closer you get to zero added sugars, the better.

You should also try to limit added sodium, also common in processed food. According to the Institute of Medicine, the average adult requires about 1,250 milligrams of sodium per day. Unfortunately, the typical Western diet delivers from 2,300 to 4,000 mg. There is a useful rule of thumb you can apply to help you keep your sodium down. Simply make sure that any packaged product you purchase has fewer milligrams of sodium than it has calories. That will save you from some whopper choices. For example, one serving of Campbell's refried beans contains 690 milligrams of sodium compared to a modest 80 calories. Or how about Healthy Choice vegetable soup, with 480 milligrams of sodium and 125 calories? Is this really a healthy choice?

Not-So-Healthy Foods—A Reminder

While planning meals, you should keep in mind the facts about a group of foods that even most vegetarians think are good for your health. We covered some of these in previous chapters, but let's look at them in the context of your personal choices. They are milk, yogurt, granola, olive oil, cheese, and fish. After being told by almost everyone for your entire life that these foods are good for you, it is certainly understandable that leaving them out of your diet might be difficult. Maybe some of this information will help.

Milk. As Dr. Campbell says in the movie *Forks over Knives*, cow's milk is nature's most perfect food—for baby cows, not for humans. Humans are the only species that drinks the milk of another species and the only species that drinks any milk at all after weaning. As you learned in the first part of the book, cow's milk contains casein, which is associated with cancer, and it has no fiber. It's also loaded with cholesterol and derives around 35 percent or more of its calories from fat.

Yogurt. Yogurt is a dairy product produced by the bacterial fermentation of milk. Though widely promoted as a healthy product that contains calcium and many vitamins, it also contains the same animal protein as milk and is associated with the same issues. It has no fiber and no phytonutrients that will help protect you against chronic disease. It is not plant-based and should not be included in your health-promoting diet.

Granola. How could granola not be good for you? Two reasons: added sugar and too much fat. Remember, you're looking for an average of less than 20 percent of your calories from fat, and you're looking for near zero added sugar. Using nutritiondata.com, we found that one serving of a homemade granola cereal contains 24 grams of sugar and a whopping 264 calories from fat, accounting for 44 percent of the total of 597 calories per serving.

Olive oil. People are always shocked to learn that olive oil is not a healthy food, but the truth is all oil derives 100 percent of its calories from fat. Your body does need fat, just as it needs carbohydrates and protein, and it gets just the right amount of all three from fruits, vegetables, grains, legumes, nuts, and seeds. As Dr. and Mrs. Esselstyn say, "You don't need oil for cooking. You can use almost any liquid—even beer or wine."[297] An optimal diet delivers less than 20 percent of its calories from fat, so choosing to use oil makes coming anywhere close to that number very difficult.

A Quick Glance at Six Not-So-Healthy Foods

Food Item	Calories from Fat (%)
Whole milk	49
Plain yogurt	47
Granola cereal	44
Olive oil	100
Cheese (American)	75
Fish (salmon)	51

All of these foods are much higher in fat than the 20 percent goal, all contain saturated fat, and most contain too much sodium and cholesterol.

If you choose to make these foods a significant part of your diet, you will have trouble achieving the health benefits that you may be seeking.

Source: NutritionData.com (details may vary based on brand chosen).

Cheese. Cheese is the most universally accepted animal product by people who consider themselves vegetarian. But cheese is not a vegetable and shares many more characteristics with meat than it does with spinach. As reported by Dr. Fuhrman in *Eat to Live*, its consumption per capita in the United States increased 140 percent between 1970 and 1996 to make it the primary source of saturated fat in our diet.[298] It is touted as being a healthy product and a good source of protein and calcium. Sadly, it has also become an integral part of every kids' menu. Cheese is not good for you, and it's not good for your children; it contains too much fat, too much cholesterol, and too much animal protein.

Fish. While fish does contain the healthy omega-3 fatty acids that our bodies need, it also contains the fat, cholesterol, animal protein, and pollutants that our bodies don't need. Do yourself and your planet a favor, and find another source for your omega-3s—flaxseed and walnuts, for example.

Nutritional Supplements: Who Needs Them?

Some of the doctors and other experts who have had success in promoting vibrant health with a plant-based diet disagree about the value of supplements. Although most agree that the majority of vitamin supplements sold today are nearly worthless and some are even dangerous, some advocate the use of supplements more than others. Dr. Neal Barnard makes an essential point: "Our bodies are designed to extract vitamins and minerals from foods. The tablets of vitamin E, beta-carotene, and the like that are sold in drug stores and health food stores greatly exceed normal quantities. In addition, these single antioxidants do not begin to match what nature offers in vegetables, fruits, and other plants."[299]

Dr. Campbell agrees: "Because nutrition operates as an infinitely complex biochemical system involving thousands of chemicals and thousands of effects on your health, it makes little or no sense that isolated nutrients taken as supplements can substitute for whole foods. Supplements will not lead to long-lasting health and may cause unforeseen side effects."[300]

Everyone must make up her own mind about where she is going to get all of the essential nutrients she needs. For myself, I have chosen to take the bottom-line advice of Dr. Campbell: "Daily supplements of vitamin B12, and perhaps vitamin D for people who spend most of their time indoors and/or live in the northern climates, are encouraged."[301]

Ordering Healthy Meals in Restaurants

Most food you find on a restaurant menu is woefully lacking in nutrients and contains far too much fat, salt, oil, white flour, and/or animal protein. Despite that, it's not that difficult to order a healthy meal while eating away from home. Creating healthy options can actually be a fun adventure. First, seek out restaurants that are likely to have some healthy foods in the kitchen. Asian restaurants will probably be your best bet. They may not have the healthy entrée items on the menu, but they will be able to put together a healthy option at your request. Italian, Indian, Mexican, and Middle Eastern restaurants are also good options. Once you have chosen the restaurant, follow these recommended steps:

1. Scan the menu, identifying what kinds of whole foods they have in the kitchen. Note the vegetables or grains they are serving with each entrée, and take a look at the side orders that they offer. Also, check to see if there is a "vegetable of the day."

2. Select an entree that features healthy whole foods, and modify it. As mentioned earlier, I frequently order the Tiger Shrimp entrée at one favorite restaurant and tell them to "hold the shrimp" and add extra vegetables and seaweed. The price usually totals half of the listed price for the shrimp entrée.

3. Ask if the chef can create a vegetable plate for you, and request that he or she use no oil, salt, butter, or cheese in the preparation. This way, the chef can be creative and can also have the freedom to select items they have in the kitchen.

4. Look for side orders on the menu. At one local restaurant, I frequently order a side of black beans and rice with a triple order of the vegetable of the day (usually broccoli or green beans). At $1.50 per side, this works out to $6.00 for a very nutritious, delicious, and filling meal (menu entrées average $18.00).

5. Order a huge salad, and add items like beans or cooked vegetables and maybe a side of whole-grain rice or whole-grain pasta to help fill you up. Ask for a dressing like balsamic vinegar or lemon juice on the side. Remember, the salad dressing alone can contain more calories than all other ingredients in the salad combined.

6. If four of you are dining together and one or two are meat eaters, consider ordering one full entrée with grilled fish, and add several sides to suit your personal tastes. Then eat family

style, with everyone eating a much smaller portion of the rich, not-so-healthy entrée—treating the "main" course as a side dish. This should satisfy those who feel that they must have their animal protein.

A word of caution: many restaurants today have the token vegetarian entrée listed on the menu. But as you now know, just because it is vegetarian doesn't mean it is necessarily a healthy choice. You're probably better off creating your own entrée and being very specific about how you want it—leaving out the white flour, oil, salt, and cheese that you will frequently find in the vegetarian entrée. For example, a typical pasta primavera will have lots of white flour pasta; precious few vegetables; and a thick, rich, creamy sauce that probably derives over 50 percent of its calories from fat. Try ordering an appetizer portion of the pasta (preferably whole-grain) with the sauce on the side. Ask them to bring all the vegetables by themselves on a plate, making sure that they add enough vegetables to fill the plate.

If you dine out often, the staff at your favorite local restaurants will enjoy creating entrees for you or will happily prepare one of your favorites every time you dine with them. Most important, dining out should be fun, your meals should be delicious and satisfying, and you should not have to compromise your healthy diet in the process. Just be creative and courteous while clearly describing exactly what you want.

Finding Healthy Options While Traveling

If possible, seek out local restaurants and follow the above guidelines. Otherwise, you can usually create a pretty healthy meal at many of the national chains such as Applebee's, Olive Garden, and Chili's. At these restaurants, follow the same general guidelines as for the local restaurants. At Subway, for instance, you can create your own vegetable sandwich. The following are some healthy snack ideas for the airplane, car, or train.

- Pack easy-to-eat foods like apples, oranges, raisins, carrot sticks, bananas, and nuts in your bag.
- Eat the healthy fruit-nuts-celery-carrots portion of the served lunch on the plane, and offer the remaining not-so-healthy items to the person seated next to you.
- If you have layovers at major airports, you can frequently find healthy food possibilities at the Asian and Mexican restaurants within the airport.
- Pack your own breakfast, lunch, or dinner, and put it in your backpack. My whole-grain spinach-stuffed pita with hummus, avocado, and olive is my favorite lunch to pack when I'm out sailing for the day.

Healthy Tips for Social or Business Occasions

You might be wondering what you will do while entertaining or when attending parties or banquets or having meals at a friend's home. What you do in these situations depends on how well you know the people. If it is a private home, explain to the host in advance that you are on a restricted diet. Explain nicely that you would like to forgo the animal-protein entrée and load up on whatever plant-based options he or she might have. Stress that there is no need to prepare anything special for you in advance. Here are five helpful tips for eating at these kinds of social functions:

1. Sometimes you may be able to select a customized healthier option in advance; a banquet may have a vegan option, for example.

2. Before leaving for the function, have a healthy snack at home so that you will not be hungry when you arrive.

3. During cocktail hour, load up on the healthy hors d'oeuvre items before sitting down to dinner.

4. If the dinner is buffet style, no problem; just load up on what you want, and no one will notice anything unusual.

5. If the hostess is serving your plate, quietly explain that your doctor has you on a special diet and that you would like to forgo the entree and add more vegetables or salad items to your plate. The less said, the better.

Finally, above all, employ courtesy and clarity. Bon appetit!

Dealing with Family and Roommates

A very important part of the adventure before you is dealing with the people with whom you share food. The sharing of food together has been an integral part of human nature since the beginning of time, and no one wants to sacrifice against his or her will. Let's look at some tips for handling three categories of people you may eat with: spouses, children, and others who might be living with you.

The spouse or significant other is by far the most important person. When you make a major change in the way you are eating, you are affecting a large portion of the time you spend together. And your spouse may very well be the person who does all the shopping and cooking. Ultimately, this new adventure will be much more rewarding if you are both on the same page. Hence, you should do all that you can to start this journey together. Maybe both of you have health issues that could be improved by a healthier diet, or you both simply want to lose weight.

Dr. Esselstyn has made involving the spouse a required part of his heart disease–reversal program at the Cleveland Clinic. He will not accept a married patient for the program unless he is joined by his spouse at the initial counseling sessions. So what if neither of you has any health issues? What if you are just convinced that this is the way you want to go and you would very much like for your spouse to join you? You might try to gently help your spouse reach your level of understanding of these powerful nutritional truths. Share reading material that you feel might suit her style. Always be respectful, never condescending, and do your best to help her understand why you feel so strongly about your new dietary regimen. In the end, a delicately balanced combination of listening, supporting, loving, understanding, and caring will be the most convincing.

Then there are your children, who may have come to believe that chicken nuggets, burgers, and fries are the primary food groups. In case anyone is fooled by the idea that all chicken is healthier than red meat, consider the following observation by Eric Schlosser in *Fast Food Nation*: "A chemical analysis of [Chicken] McNuggets by a researcher at Harvard Medical School found that their 'fatty acid profile' more closely resembled beef than poultry . . . Today, Chicken McNuggets are wildly popular among young children—and contain twice as much fat per ounce as a hamburger."[302]

The earlier you start your kids on the right road, the better. As mentioned previously, it is also essential that their parents eat the same diet to model healthy eating. After reading Joel Fuhrman's *Disease-Proof Your Child*, my son, who is the father of four young children, immediately removed all the unhealthy items from his house. The kids were young enough that they accepted the new routine with no problems. If you're dealing with children twelve years old or older, however, the change is going to be more difficult. Your likelihood of success will depend on your level of commitment to making this work. Just keep in the back of your mind that someday they will greatly appreciate the fact that their parents were leaders in the great food revolution of the twenty-first century.

You may also have roommates—family or friends—who share your living space. This situation is far less challenging for obvious reasons.

Certainly, you should try to help them understand the benefits of the diet you have adopted. But if they don't, just pretend that you are living alone as far as eating is concerned. You can still eat together, but you may have to obtain or prepare your food separately. Take care of your own needs, and never criticize. If they ever want your help or advice, they will ask for it.

Recommended Books
with Healthy Recipes and Meal Plans

A key part of making the switch is using proven healthy recipes to help ease the transition to this new way of eating. The following books not only contain helpful meal plans and healthy, delicious recipes; they also provide the reader with additional information about this powerful health regimen.

1. *Eat to Live* by Joel Fuhrman. This is one of the first books I read on the optimal diet, and it is highly recommended. Dr. Fuhrman designed the nutrient-scoring index that is used all across the United States in the fresh produce department of Whole Foods Market.

2. *The McDougall Plan* by John McDougall and Mary A. McDougall. This is another highly recommended read for anyone interested in taking charge of his or her health. The book features a great chart in the appendix that shows the percentages of protein, carbohydrates, and fat in all kinds of food. The book also includes lots of terrific recipes.

3. *Prevent and Reverse Heart Disease* by Caldwell Esselstyn, Jr. The book begins by explaining the simplicity of a whole-foods, plant-based diet that has been proven to reverse heart disease. It contains more than 150 recipes.

4. *The Spectrum* by Dean Ornish. This is a *New York Times* bestseller that features a plant-based solution to taking charge of
   our health. Its Part II, consisting of over 100 pages, is all about
   preparing delicious and healthy meals in the kitchen. Also, visit
   www.pmri.org and www.ornishspectrum.com.

5. *No More Bull!* by Howard Lyman. This is a very entertaining
   read by a former cattle rancher turned vegan. It is a compact
   and informative source of information about the power of
   a whole-foods, plant-based diet and includes many great
   recipes.

6. *The Engine 2 Diet* by Rip Esselstyn. This is a great book for
   guys. Written by a former world-class triathlete and firefighter,
   this book helps a lot of macho men understand that the plant-
   based diet is not for sissies. About half the book is devoted to
   tasty, healthy recipes. As you may have guessed, the author's
   father is Dr. Caldwell Esselstyn, Jr., of the Cleveland Clinic.

7. *Disease-Proof Your Child* by Joel Fuhrman. This book
   helped my son make the decision to adopt this healthy diet
   completely—not so much for himself at first but for his children. It is highly recommended for parents of children of all
   ages. It contains lots of tasty and fun recipes.

In addition to these seven books, you should also visit the helpful
website of the T. Colin Campbell Foundation at TColinCampbell.org.
In October 2010, this wonderful website launched a user-generated
online recipe guide. It features only plant-based foods, and all recipes
are reviewed by Dr. Campbell's staff before they appear on the site.
Finally, you will want to order your own copy of *The China Study*.
Although it doesn't contain recipes, it does contain a very helpful
chapter outlining a series of principles for healthy eating. In addition,
you will refer to this great book often as questions come up about the
scientific legitimacy of the plant-based diet.

Easing Your Transition

During the early stages of adopting this healthy lifestyle, you may possibly experience some temporary discomfort. When you move quickly from a highly toxic diet to one of nutritional excellence, your body may go through a sort of withdrawal as it cleanses itself and adjusts to this superior way of eating. This natural detoxification may include some minor fevers and some unusual stools. Without some advance warning of this phenomenon, you might be alarmed and want to return to your old way of eating. Ride it out. Just pay attention to your body, give it the best possible foods, and the discomfort will pass.

Here are a few tips to make your life easier as you make the transition:

1. Keep it simple. Whether for breakfast, lunch, or dinner, don't be reluctant to eat something simple like an apple, a pear, or a plate of veggies with homemade hummus.
2. Eat when hungry. Begin eating early in the morning; then eat when you're hungry after that. You should never have to suffer. Keep those healthy snacks nearby when there are long stretches between meals.
3. Cook in multiday batches. Most of my in-home lunches or dinners contain a side order of legumes, wild rice, and/or brown rice. Try making up enough for a few days; then package the rice and beans in single-serving containers. Using this method, I can prepare my typical lunch of 600 calories in five minutes. I just add other whole plant foods such as mushrooms, olives, tomatoes, carrots, avocados, broccoli, spinach, eggplant, and hummus.
4. Keep only healthy snacks in your home. We all get hungry between meals and don't have the time to prepare something to eat. Keep healthy snack choices on hand for those times: grapes or other fruit, carrots, celery, broccoli, and nuts. (Go easy on the nuts unless you're a lean athlete who burns many calories.)

5. Avoid fake meats. The whole idea is to start new habits to give you the health-promoting power of whole plant foods. Meat substitutes are highly processed, usually have way too much sodium, and tend to remind you of the foods that you used to crave. Embrace your new diet, and develop a new list of your favorite health-promoting foods. If you don't learn to love this new way of eating, you will have difficulty sticking with it.

6. Get a healthy start each day. By starting the day with fruit, you're getting a jump start on your day with some of nature's most perfect foods. Eat it alone or with whole-grain cereal.

Answering the Inevitable Questions

When you make a lifestyle change like this, you will be asked many questions—from friends, family, coworkers, casual acquaintances, golf buddies, or fellow members of your club or church. There are two questions that you will hear most: (1) Why are you eating this way? (2) Where do you get your protein?

They may also follow up with queries like, "Do you mean to say that you don't even eat cheese? Or fish?" They may ask the same question in many different ways, and sometimes you'll sense hostility in their questions. Generally, this negativity stems from frustration about aspects of their own lives: their health, their weight, or their inability to adopt a superior diet. They may ask if you're eating this way for health, religious, environmental, ethical, or other reasons.

You can answer the second question, about protein, with the facts from Chapter 3. But the way you answer the first question depends on the relationship you have with the person asking. The following are a few examples of how you might want to answer someone who has asked you, "Why are you eating this way?"

- A stranger sitting next to you on an airplane asks the question. Your answer might be something as simple as "Doctor's orders."

- A coworker has noticed what you're eating each day at lunch and is curious. You might say something like, "Well, I started out for health reasons a few years ago but have since learned about how many important things in this world are greatly affected by what we eat." If the coworker wants to hear more, he will ask a follow-up question.

- One of your old friends comes up to you in private after your twenty-fifth high school reunion, comments on how good you're looking, and asks about why you only ate the veggies from the buffet. In this case, your answer might be something a little bit deeper. "You know, Tom, awhile back I became aware of the enormous impact that what we eat has on many aspects of our entire world. And not having *given back* much during the first forty years of my life, I decided that eating this way would enable me to effortlessly do some wonderful things for my health, for my family, for my fellow man, and for the planet—all at the same time." Maybe he'll invite you to dinner and have a few more probing questions about what you're eating and why.

During my early years of learning the big-picture truths about nutrition, John Robbins helped bring that picture into focus for me. These words from his *Food Revolution* come to mind now as I reflect on the beauty and simplicity of this wonderful way of eating that enables me to live in harmony with planet Earth: "To me it is deeply moving that the same food choices that give us the best chance to eliminate world hunger are also those that take the least toll on the environment, contribute most to our long-term health, are the safest, and are also far and away the most compassionate toward our fellow creatures."[303]

Keep these words in mind as you begin your journey to vibrant health and beyond.

And, as you begin that journey, we would like to help you. For frequently updated information, tips and guidelines—please visit our website at HealthyEatingHealthyWorld.com, which also serves as the home of my blog. For help with our 4-Leaf Program, you can go directly to 4LeafProgram.com.

Finally, if you have questions or comments for either of us, you can email me directly at jmh@jmorrishicks.com or to my son and co-writer at jason@jstanfieldhicks.com. We look forward to hearing from you and hearing about your progress as we work together to make things better for our planet, ourselves, and for all of those who follow us. Good luck and God bless you.

"Patience and perseverance have a magical effect before which difficulties disappear and obstacles vanish."

—John Quincy Adams

11

A RETURN TO HARMONY

"Faced with what is right, to leave it undone shows a lack of courage."

—Confucius

The world's scientists have recorded over 50,000 vertebrate species on planet Earth, including some 5,500 species of mammals.[304] Other vertebrates include fish, reptiles, birds, and amphibians. Beyond the vertebrates are about 1 million named species of insects, and scientists estimate that millions more are yet to be discovered. For eons, all of those species lived in harmony with each other and their natural environment—until recently. Over the past century, the human species has distinguished itself as the only one that is not living in harmony with the rest of the planet.

What is needed to correct this problem is *a blinding flash of the obvious*. One of the geniuses of the modern era, Albert Einstein, said it best: "Nothing will benefit human health and increase chances of survival for life on earth as much as the evolution to a vegetarian diet."

Deep down inside, we may have all sensed for some time that something was terribly wrong with our way of life and its host of negative consequences for our planet. We just haven't had a clear understanding of what it was, how it got that way, or what—if anything—we could do about it. I hope your vision of what's wrong with this picture is more in focus now that you better understand the staggering damage that has resulted from our way of eating. Returning to a more natural diet for our species won't solve all our problems overnight, but it will be a pretty good start.

In a mere blink in the lifespan of our planet, we got into this mess; maybe we can get out of it in even less time. If all of this makes sense to you, then it's time to come to grips with what it means. With this new knowledge comes responsibility. Now that you know how to easily solve the health-care crisis, make tremendous environmental improvements, greatly reduce our dependence on fossil fuels, feed the hungry, and end the widespread suffering of animals, what are you going to do with that knowledge? Simply knowing something doesn't change anything or make anything better. An ancient Persian proverb states, "It is nothing for one to know something unless another knows you know it." Every single person can make a difference by actively participating in a collective *return to harmony*. Beginning with just a few people, this grassroots effort can gather momentum quickly.

How much more information do we need? When will enough informed citizens aggressively demand the changes that are so urgently needed? How many more headlines like the following one are needed to make the world's leaders acknowledge the obvious solution to so many interconnected world issues?

Diabetes Cases May Triple by 2050

This was the front-page headline in *USA Today* on October, 22, 2010. Citing a new report from the CDC, the article says, "[O]ne in ten U.S. adults has diabetes now. The prevalence is expected to rise sharply over the next 40 years with as many as one in three having the disease, primarily type 2 diabetes, according to the report, published in the journal *Population Health Metrics*."[305] The next evening on *Saturday Night Live*, Seth Meyers commented on that same CDC report during the Weekend Update portion of the show, saying, "That can't be too surprising—for a country that uses fried chicken as bread."[306] This kind of humor just reinforces the fact that everyone suspects what a toxic diet we're consuming. We're not just eating too much food; we're eating the wrong food.

This type of runaway growth of such an easily preventable (or reversible) disease is simply unacceptable. Our extended health-care system continues to talk about managing diseases like diabetes but fails to acknowledge what a handful of highly regarded scientists and medical doctors have known for a long time: the vast majority of all of our health-care issues are food-driven. And the answer is right under our noses.

We can simply change what we put in our mouths every day. By eating a health-promoting diet, we have the power to reverse many personal and worldwide problems. When enough people participate in changing their eating habits, the markets will respond, and the movement will gain momentum. With a solid understanding of the enormity of what is at stake, you can make a difference. Even better, you can help others understand as well. Are you going to keep this knowledge to yourself?

Obviously, you can start with sharing what you've learned with your own family, beginning with your children. By helping your children adopt this powerful way of eating, you will be ensuring not only their lifelong health but also the health of future generations of your family. Beyond your children and other close relatives, you can share your newfound knowledge with other people you care about. Without being preachy or proselytizing, you can share what you know with those who show an interest. They will pass the good word along.

You might also think about starting a study group in your community, writing to your legislators at the state and federal level, submitting articles to local newspapers, hosting speakers in your community, or organizing a proactive task force to spread the word on your college campus. Or you can aim lower. Help just three people understand what you have learned about the *world-changing power of plant-based nutrition,* and influence them to make some changes in their own lives.

If each person reaches just three people over the course of a year, we could dramatically change the world in less than five years. This is how to launch a grassroots revolution in health-care and so much more—by spreading the information to as many people as possible. Then, we hope, we will live to see the day that our highly inefficient, destructive, and disease-promoting Western diet is simply "not cool" anymore—much like cigarette smoking. How many people do you need to start a revolution? History tells us that you don't need as many as you might think—a lot closer to 10 percent of the population than 50 percent.

In a world full of sick, obese, or starving people, suffering animals and rapidly disappearing natural resources; how can we possibly not come together and end all of this madness once and for all? Given what you now know—if you don't take action—what will you tell your adult grandchildren someday when they ask why you didn't?

Ultimately, your decision is a simple matter of health, hope, and harmony. As each of us begins to take charge of his or her own health, we simultaneously plant the seeds of hope, accelerating the pace with which the human race can return to living in harmony with nature. Since we consider ourselves smarter than all the other creatures, we should be able to figure out how to make our world a better place. The time for that action is now.

"You may never know what results come of your action, but if you do nothing, there will be no result."

—Mahatma Gandhi

ABOUT THE AUTHOR

A former management consultant and senior corporate executive with Ralph Lauren in New York, J. Morris Hicks has always focused on the "big picture" when analyzing any issue. In 2002, after becoming curious about our "optimal diet," he began an intensive study of what we eat from a global perspective—discovering many startling issues and opportunities along the way.

Leveraging his expertise in making complex things simple, he is now helping people everywhere understand the staggering "big picture" impact of how our food choices affect so many crucial aspects of life as we know it—beginning with our own health and the out-of-control cost of health care. In his new career as a writer, speaker, blogger, and consultant, he is now working to improve the global human feeding model—all aimed at promoting health, hope, and harmony on planet Earth.

He holds a BS in Industrial Engineering from Auburn University and an MBA from the University of Hawaii. In 2009, he earned a Certificate in Plant-Based Nutrition from the T. Colin Campbell Foundation and Cornell University. Since 2003, he has resided in the seaside village of Stonington, Connecticut.

NOTES

1. www.nutritiondata.com.
2. Bruce Bartlett, "Health Care: Costs and Reform," *Forbes*, July 3, 2009, http://www.forbes.com/2009/07/02/health-care-costs-opinions-columnists-reform.html.
3. www.libraryindex.com/pages/1226/.
4. Denise Grady, "Obesity Rates Keep Rising, Troubling Health Officials," *New York Times*, August 4, 2010, A11.
5. World Health Organization, "Obesity and Overweight," 2003, http://www.who.int/hpr/NPH/docs/gs_obesity.pdf.
6. Centers for Disease Control and Prevention, "Heart Disease Facts," December 21, 2010, http://www.cdc.gov/heartdisease/facts.htm.
7. Nicholas Bakalar, "Vital Statistics; Diabetes: A State-by-State Breakdown," *New York Times*, October 13, 2009, http://query.nytimes.com/gst/fullpage.html?res=9504E1D91F3BF930A25753C1A96F9C8B63.
8. N. R. Kleinfield, "Diabetes and Its Awful Toll Quietly Emerge as a Crisis," *New York Times*, January 9, 2006, http://www.nytimes.com/2006/01/09/nyregion/nyregionspecial5/09diabetes.html?pagewanted=1&_r=1.
9. Ibid.
10. John Robbins, *Healthy at 100: The Scientifically Proven Secrets of the World's Healthiest and Longest-Lived Peoples* (New York: Random House, 2006), 57.
11. Joel Fuhrman, *Eat to Live: The Revolutionary Formula for Fast and Sustained Weight Loss* (Boston: Little, Brown, 2003), 118.
12. Christopher McDougall, "The Men Who Live Forever," *Men's Health*, June 28, 2006, http://www.menshealth.com/fitness/longevity.

13. Harvey Levenstein, "Food and Diet," in *The Oxford Companion to United States History*, ed. Paul S. Boyer (New York: Oxford University Press, 2001), 272.

14. Humane Society of the United States, "Farm Animal Statistics: Meat Consumption," November 30, 2006, http://www.humanesociety.org/news/resources/research/stats_meat_consumption.html.

15. Joel Fuhrman, *Eat to Live*, 80.

16. Eric Schlosser, *Fast Food Nation: The Dark Side of the All-American Meal* (New York: Harper Perennial, 2005), 229.

17. Douglas J. Lisle and Alan Goldhamer, *The Pleasure Trap: Mastering the Force That Undermines Health and Happiness* (Summertown, TN: Healthy Living Publications, 2003), 9–10.

18. Ibid., 42.

19. T. Colin Campbell, *The China Study: The Most Comprehensive Study of Nutrition Ever Conducted and the Startling Implications for Diet, Weight Loss and Long-term Health* (Dallas: BenBella Books, 2005), 234.

20. John A. McDougall, *The McDougall Program for a Healthy Heart: A Lifesaving Approach to Preventing and Treating Heart Disease* (New York: Plume, 1998), 11.

21. Nancy J. Nelson, "Migrant Studies Aid the Search for Factors Linked to Breast Cancer Risk," *Journal of the National Cancer Institute* 98, no. 7 (April 2006): 436.

22. Ibid.

23. Ibid.

24. BBC News, "Chinese Concern at Obesity Surge," October 12, 2004, http://news.bbc.co.uk/2/hi/asia-pacific/3737162.stm.

25. Campbell, *The China Study*, 71 and 149.

26. World Health Organization, "Global Strategy on Diet, Physical Activity and Health," 2009, http://www.who.int/dietphysicalactivity/strategy/eb11344/strategy_english_web.pdf.

27. Esselstyn, in lectures and videos.

28. Campbell, *The China Study*, 129.

29. Dean Ornish, *Dr. Dean Ornish's Program for Reversing Heart Disease* (New York: Ballantine, 1996), 14.

30. Campbell, *The China Study*, 130.

31. Neal D. Barnard, *Dr. Neal Barnard's Program for Reversing Diabetes: The Scientifically Proven System for Reversing Diabetes without Drugs* (New York: Rodale, 2007), 11.

32. James W. Anderson and Kyleen Ward, "High-Carbohydrate, High-Fiber Diets for Insulin-Treated Men with Diabetes Mellitus," *American Journal of Clinical Nutrition* 32 (November 1979): 2312–321.

33. Barnard, *Dr. Neal Barnard's Program for Reversing Diabetes*, 17.

34. Campbell, *The China Study*, 5.

35. Campbell, a direct quote in private.

36. Ibid.

37. Ibid., 6.

38. Jane E. Brody, "Huge Study of Diet Indicts Fat and Meat," *New York Times*, May 8, 1990, http://www.nytimes.com/1990/05/08/science/huge-study-of-diet-indicts-fat-and-meat.html?src=pm.

39. Campbell, *The China Study*, xi.

40. Ibid., 110.

41. William C. Roberts, "We Think We Are One, We Act as If We Are One, but We Are Not One," *American Journal of Cardiology* 66, no. 10 (1990): 896.

42. Joel Fuhrman, *Eat to Live*, 45.

43. Campbell, *The China Study*, 224.

44. Bartlett, "Health Care: Costs and Reform."

45. Campbell, *The China Study*, 346–47.

46. McDougall, *The McDougall Program for a Healthy Heart*, 10.

47. Caldwell Esselstyn, Jr., *Prevent and Reverse Heart Disease: The Revolutionary, Scientifically Proven, Nutrition-Based Cure* (New York: Penguin, 2007), 98.

48. William F. Enos, Robert H. Holmes, and James Beyer, "Coronary Disease among United States Soldiers Killed in Action in Korea," *Journal of the American Medical Association* 152, no. 12 (1953): 1090–93.

49. Steve Sternberg, "Russert death shows heart attack not easy to predict," *USA Today*, June 16, 2008.

50. Campbell, *The China Study*, 123 (emphasis in original).

51. Campbell, *The China Study*, 114-15.

52. Ornish, *Dr. Dean Ornish's Program for Reversing Heart Disease*, 286.

53. Ibid., 255.

54. Campbell, *The China Study*, 123.

55. Furhman, *Eat to Live*, 146.

56. Barnard, *Dr. Neal Barnard's Program for Reversing Diabetes*, 43.

57. Caldwell Esselstyn, Jr., "Is the Present Therapy for Coronary Artery Disease the Radical Mastectomy of the Twenty-First Century?" *American Journal of Cardiology* 106, no. 6 (September 2010): 902–4.

58. Esselstyn, *Prevent and Reverse Heart Disease*, 98.

59. Campbell, *The China Study*, 145.

60. Kleinfield, "Diabetes and Its Awful Toll Quietly Emerge as a Crisis."

61. Campbell, *The China Study*, 146.

62. Kleinfield, "Diabetes and Its Awful Toll Quietly Emerge as a Crisis."

63. Campbell, *The China Study*, 152.

64. Barnard, *Dr. Neal Barnard's Program for Reversing Diabetes*, 14.

65. Ibid.

66. Ornish, *Dr. Dean Ornish's Program for Reversing Heart Disease.*

67. Fuhrman, *Eat to Live*, 159.

68. Ornish, *Dr. Dean Ornish's Program for Reversing Heart Disease*, xxviii–xxix.

69. Campbell, *The China Study*, 12.

70. Marilynn Marchione, "Cancer Is the World's Costliest Disease, Says American Cancer Society," Huffington Post, August 16, 2010, http://www.huffingtonpost.com/2010/08/16/cancer-is-the-worlds-cost_n_683894.html.

71. World Cancer Research Fund/American Institute for Cancer Research, *Food, Nutrition, Physical Activity, and the Prevention of Cancer: A Global Perspective* (Washington, DC: AICR, 2007), 228.

72. Fuhrman, *Eat to Live*, 81.

73. Campbell, *The China Study*, 182.

74. Ibid., 48–50, 59.

75. Campbell, *The China Study*, 182.

76. Ibid., 204.

77. Ibid., 205.

78. McDougall, *The McDougall Program for Healthy Heart*, 102.

79. Campbell, *The China Study*, 238.

80. Ibid.

81. Barnard, *Dr. Neal Barnard's Program for Reversing Diabetes*, 20–21.

82. Ornish, *Dr. Dean Ornish's Program for Reversing Heart Disease*, 250 (emphasis in original).

83. Campbell, *The China Study*, 225.

84. *Forks over Knives*, directed by Lee Fulkerson (Monica Beach Media, 2010).

85. Lea Winerman, "Workers Paying More for Health Insurance as Cash-Strapped Companies Shift Costs," *New York Times*, September 2, 2010, http://www.pbs.org/newshour/rundown/2010/09/workers-paying-more-for-health-insurance-as-cash-strapped-companies-shift-costs.html.

86. Winerman, "Workers Paying More for Health Insurance as Cash-Strapped Companies Shift Costs."

87. Carol Morello, "About 44 Million in U.S. Lived below Poverty Line in 2009, Census Data Show," *Washington Post*, September 16, 2010, http://www.washingtonpost.com/wp-dyn/content/article/2010/09/16/AR2010091602698.html.

88. Ibid.

89. "Vegetarianism in America," *Vegetarian Times*, 2008, http://www.vegetariantimes.com/features/archive_of_editorial/667.

90. John A. McDougall and Mary A. McDougall, *The McDougall Plan* (Indianapolis: New Century, 1983), 322.

91. Ornish, *Dr. Dean Ornish's Program for Reversing Heart Disease*, 251.

92. Ibid.

93. Esselstyn, *Prevent and Reverse Heart Disease*, 77.

94. McDougall and McDougall, *The McDougall Plan*, 5.

95. Barnard, *Dr. Neal Barnard's Program for Reversing Diabetes*, 66–67.

96. Fuhrman, *Eat to Live*, 137.

97. Campbell, *The China Study*, 30–31.

98. Ibid., 31.

99. McDougall and McDougall, *The McDougall Plan*, 39.

100. Barnard, *Dr. Neal Barnard's Program for Reversing Diabetes*, 47.

101. Fuhrman, *Eat to Live*, 123–24.

102. Howard F. Lyman, *No More Bull! The Mad Cowboy Targets America's Worst Enemy: Our Diet* (New York: Scribner, 2005), 41.

103. Ibid, 42.

104. Campbell, *The China Study*, 282.

105. Table adapted from George Mateljan Foundation, "How Can I Get More Omega-3 Fatty Acids in My Daily Meals?" *The World's Healthiest Foods*, www.whfoods.com/genpage.php?tname=george&dbid=75.

106. Barnard, *Dr. Neal Barnard's Program for Reversing Diabetes*, 43.

107. Fuhrman, *Eat to Live*, 84.
108. McDougall and McDougall, *The McDougall Plan*, 52.
109. Campbell, *The China Study*, 6.
110. Common domain information.
111. Barnard, *Dr. Neal Barnard's Program for Reversing Diabetes*, 70.
112. McDougall, *The McDougall Program for a Healthy Heart*, 121.
113. USDA Economic Research Service, "Chicken Consumption Continues Longrun Rise," *AmberWaves*, April 2006, http://www.ers.usda.gov/amberwaves/april06/findings/chicken.htm.
114. Mark Bittman, "Rethinking the Meat-Guzzler," *New York Times*, January 27, 2008, http://www.nytimes.com/2008/0½27/weekinreview/27bittman.html.
115. Ibid.
116. Jonathan Safran Foer, *Eating Animals* (New York: Little, Brown, 2009), 144.
117. Schlosser, *Fast Food Nation*, 136.
118. Anna Lappé, *Diet for a Hot Planet: The Climate Crisis at the End of Your Fork and What You Can Do about It* (New York: Bloomsbury, 2010), 21.
119. Foer, *Eating Animals*, 109.
120. Ibid., 170.
121. Food and Agricultural Organization of the United Nations, *Livestock's Long Shadow: Environmental Issues and Options* (Rome: FAO, 2006), xx.
122. Ibid., 74.
123. Ibid, Executive Summary, xxi.
124. Ibid.
125. John Robbins, *Diet for a New America: How Your Food Choices Affect Your Health, Happiness, and the Future of Life on Earth* (Tiburon, CA: H J Kramer, 1987), 358.
126. "Land Degradation," University of Michigan Global Change Program, January 4, 2010, http://www.globalchange.umich.edu/globalchange2/current/lectures/land_deg/land_deg.html.
127. David Pimentel, "Soil Erosion: A Food and Environmental Threat," *Environment, Development and Sustainability* 8, no. 1 (2006)
128. Howard F. Lyman, *Mad Cowboy: Plain Truth from the Cattle Rancher Who Won't Eat Meat* (New York: Touchstone, 1998), 147.
129. Ibid., 145–46.
130. Robbins, *Diet for a New America*, 360.

131. FAO, *Livestock's Long Shadow*, 82, 112, 114, Executive Summary xxi.
132. A. R. Ravishankara, John S. Daniel, and Robert W. Portmann, "Nitrous Oxide (N2O): The Dominant Ozone-Depleting Substance Emitted in the 21st Century," *Science*, October 2, 2009, 123–25.
133. Lyman, *Mad Cowboy*, 127.
134. FAO, *Livestock's Long Shadow*, 104.
135. Vital Water Graphics, An Overview of the State of the World's Fresh and Marine Waters—2nd Edition—2008. Executive Summary, #3. This is a joint publication of the United Nations Environment Programme (UNEP) and its collaborating centre UNEP/ GRID-Arendal in Norway. It is published as part of UNEP's global water policy and strategy. www.unep.org/dewa/vitalwater/ article186.html
136. Fred Pearce, *When the Rivers Run Dry: Water—The Defining Crisis of the Twenty-First Century* (Boston: Beacon Press, 2006), 4.
137. Lyman, *Mad Cowboy*, 132–33.
138. Pearce, *When the Rivers Run Dry*, 38.
139. Tom Aldridge and Herb Schlubach, "Water Requirements for Food Production," *Soil and Water* 38 (Fall 1978).
140. Lyman, *Mad Cowboy*, 132 (emphasis in original).
141. Elizabeth Limbach, "Eating for the Environment," *Good Times*, April 14, 2010, http://www.goodtimessantacruz.com/good-times-cover-stories/1027-eating-for-the-environment.html.
142. Foer, *Eating Animals*, 174.
143. David Kirby, *Animal Factory: The Looming Threat of Industrial Pig, Dairy and Poultry Farms to Humans and the Environment* (New York, St. Martin's Press, 2010), xv.
144. http://www.nrdc.org/water/pollution/ffarms.asp.
145. Jeff Tietz, "Boss Hog," *Rolling Stone*, December 14, 2006, http:// wannaveg.com/2007/01/15/rolling-stone-boss-hog/.
146. Charles Duhigg, "Health Ills Abound as Farm Runoff Fouls Wells," *New York Times*, September 18, 2009, A1.
147. Ibid.
148. Foer, *Eating Animals*, 173.
149. Doreen Carvajal and Stephen Castle, "A U.S. Hog Giant Transforms Eastern Europe," *New York Times*, May 5, 2009, http:// www.nytimes.com/2009/05/06/business/global/06smithfield .html?pagewanted=1&_r=1.

150. Center for International Environmental Law (CIEL), "What Is Biodiversity and Why Is It Important?" http://www.ciel.org/Biodiversity/WhatIsBiodiversity.html.

151. FAO, *Livestock's Long Shadow*, 182.

152. Ibid., 215.

153. CIEL, "What Is Biodiversity and Why Is It Important?"

154. Ibid.

155. John Robbins, *The Food Revolution: How Your Diet Can Help Save Your Life and Our World* (San Francisco: Conari Press, 2001), 255, 257.

156. Ibid., 269.

157. FAO, *Livestock's Long Shadow*, 205.

158. Bruce Monger, "Principles in Practice: Food Production and Environmental Concerns," lecture 2, course in Cornell's Plant-Based Nutrition certificate program.

159. Ibid.

160. Ibid.

161. Robbins, *The Food Revolution*, 232–33.

162. Rick Jervis and Kevin Johnson, "BP Works on More Secure Well Cap," *USA Today*, July 12, 2010, http://www.usatoday.com/news/nation/2010-07-11-oilspill-cap_N.htm.

163. Energy Information Administration (EIA).

164. Jeff Rubin, *Why Your World Is about to Get a Whole Lot Smaller: Oil and the End of Globalization* (New York: Random House, 2009), 158.

165. Ibid., 223.

166. Julian Cribb, *The Coming Famine: The Global Food Crisis and What We Can Do to Avoid It* (Berkeley and Los Angeles: University of California Press, 2010), 119.

167. Bill McKibben, *Deep Economy: Economics as If the World Mattered* (Oxford: Oneworld, 2007), 64.

168. Rubin, *Why Your World Is about to Get a Whole Lot Smaller*, 220.

169. Lyman, *Mad Cowboy*, 126.

170. Bittman, "Rethinking the Meat-Guzzler."

171. FAO, "Framework for Calculating Fossil Fuel Use in Livestock Systems," http://www.fao.org/agriculture/lead/tools/fossil/ru.

172. Robbins, *The Food Revolution*, 266.

173. Lyman, *Mad Cowboy*, 126.

174. Limbach, "Eating for the Environment."

175. U.S. Energy Information Administration.
176. Ibid.
177. Rubin, *Why Your World Is about to Get a Whole Lot Smaller*, 104.
178. "Ethanol's Grocery Bill," *Wall Street Journal*, June 3, 2009, A13.
179. Ibid.
180. Elisabeth Rosenthal, "U.N. Says Biofuel Subsidies Raise Food Bill and Hunger," *New York Times*, October 7, 2008, http://www.nytimes.com/2008/10/08/world/europe/08italy.html.
181. Ibid.
182. Cribb, *The Coming Famine*, 124.
183. Rubin, *Why Your World Is about to Get a Whole Lot Smaller*, 100.
184. Ibid., 220.
185. McKibben, *Deep Economy*, 66.
186. Cribb, *The Coming Famine*, 10.
187. Schlosser, *Fast Food Nation*, 230.
188. Julian Borger, "Feed the World? We Are Fighting a Losing Battle, UN Admits," *Guardian*, February 26, 2008, http://www.guardian.co.uk/environment/2008/feb/26/food.unitednations. http://www.nytimes.com/2008/10/08/world/europe/08italy.html.
189. Neil MacFarquhar, "UN Raises Concerns as Global Food Prices Jump," *New York Times*, September 4, 2010, A4.
190. Jean Ziegler, Right to Food website, www.righttofood.org.
191. Jean Ziegler, *L'Empire de la honte* (Livre de Poche, 2007), 130.
192. David Pimentel, "Principles in Practice: Food Production and Environmental Concerns," lecture 1, course in Cornell's Plant-Based Nutrition certificate program.
193. Richard L. Lobb, "Green Revolution," in *Encyclopedia of Food and Culture*, ed. Solomon H. Katz and William Woys Weaver (New York: Charles Scribner's, 2003), http://www.encyclopedia.com/topic/Green_Revolution.aspx.
194. Ibid.
195. Robbins, *Diet for a New America*, 352.
196. Ibid.
197. U.S. Census Bureau, "World POPClock Projection," http://www.census.gov/ipc/www/popclockworld.html.
198. www.ers.usda.gov/publications/aer823/aer823c.pdf.
199. Mark Bittman, "Seeing a Time (Soon) When We'll All Be Dieting," *New York Times*, August 24, 2010, http://www.nytimes.com/2010/08/25/books/25book.html.

200. Rubin, *Why Your World Is about to Get a Whole Lot Smaller*, 225.
201. Pimentel, "Principles in Practice: Food Production and Environmental Concerns," lecture 1.
202. Cribb, *The Coming Famine*, 69.
203. Foer, *Eating Animals*, 73.
204. Kirby, *Animal Factory*, 33.
205. William Neuman, "Egg Farms Violated Safety Rules," *New York Times*, August 30, 2010, http://www.nytimes.com/2010/08/31/business/31eggs.html.
206. Michael Pollan, "Profiles in Courage on Animal Welfare," *New York Times*, May 29, 2006, http://pollan.blogs.nytimes.com/2006/05/29/profiles-in-courage-on-animal-welfare.
207. Jane Goodall, *Harvest for Hope: A Guide to Mindful Eating* (New York: Warner Books, 2005), 69–70.
208. Robbins, *Diet for a New America*, 63.
209. Foer, *Eating Animals*, 59–60.
210. Ibid., 60.
211. Humane Society of the United States, "The Dirty Six: The Worst Animal Practices in Agribusiness," in *Food, Inc.*, ed. Karl Weber (New York: PublicAffairs, 2009), 63.
212. Ibid., 62.
213. Ibid., 48.
214. Ibid., 48–49.
215. Ibid., 63.
216. William Neuman, "New Way to Help Chickens Cross to Other Side," *New York Times*, October 21, 2010, http://www.nytimes.com/2010/10/22/business/22chicken.html?_r=1. http://pollan.blogs.nytimes.com/2006/05/29/profiles-in-courage-on-animal-welfare.
217. Hajiba Zaaboul, "Effects of Age and Method of Castration on Performance and Stress Response of Beef Cattle," TheBeefSite.com, February 2007, http://thebeefsite.com/articles/909/effects-of-age-and-method-of-castration-on-performance-and-stress-response-of-beef-cattle.
218. Schlosser, *Fast Food Nation*, 149–50.
219. Michael Pollan, *The Omnivore's Dilemma: A Natural History of Four Meals* (New York: Penguin Press, 2006), 304.
220. Foer, *Eating Animals*, 227.
221. Robbins, *The Food Revolution*, 211.
222. Ibid., 172.

223. Kirby, *Animal Factory*, 25.
224. Tietz, "Boss Hog," http://wannaveg.com/2007/01/15/rolling-stone-boss-hog/.
225. Ibid.
226. Kirby, *Animal Factory*, 224–25.
227. Foer, *Eating Animals*, 191.
228. Ibid.
229. Robbins, *The Food Revolution*, 298.
230. Barry Estabrook, "Salmon Farms: Feedlots of the Sea," *Atlantic*, February 17, 2010, http://www.theatlantic.com/food/archive/2010/02/salmon-farms-feedlots-of-the-sea/36071.
231. Terry McCarthy, "Is Fish Farming Safe?" *Time*, November 17, 2002, http://www.time.com/time/globalbusiness/article/0,9171,391523,00.html.
232. Robbins, *The Food Revolution*, 299.
233. Foer, *Eating Animals*, 189.
234. Maggie Jones, "The Barnyard Strategist," *New York Times Magazine*, October 24, 2008, http://www.nytimes.com/2008/10/26/magazine/26animal-t.html.
235. Michael Pollan, "Profiles in Courage on Animal Welfare."
236. Foer, *Eating Animals*, 193.
237. Ibid., 148.
238. Campbell, *The China Study*, 250.
239. See Campbell, *The China Study*, 249–350.
240. Bartlett, "Health Care: Costs and Reform."
241. Ibid.
242. U.S. Department of Labor, Bureau of Labor Statistics, "Career Guide to Industries, 2010–11 Edition," February 2, 2010, http://www.bls.gov/oco/cg/cgs035.htm.
243. Marion Nestle, *Food Politics: How the Food Industry Influences Nutrition and Health* (Berkeley and Los Angeles: University of California Press, 2002), 11.
244. Ross Eisenbrey, "Health Insurance Industry Employment Outpacing Providers and All-Industry Growth Rates," Economic Policy Institute, September 18, 2007, http://www.epi.org/economic_snapshots/entry/webfeatures_snapshots_20070919.
245. John McDougall, "Real Healthcare Reform Has *Health* as the Primary Goal," *McDougall Newsletter* 8, no. 6 (June 2009), http://www.drmcdougall.com/misc/2009nl/jun/real.htm.
246. Campbell, *The China Study*, 321.

247. Ibid., 332.
248. Duff Wilson, "Harvard Medical School in Ethics Quandary," *New York Times*, March 2, 2009, http://www.nytimes.com/2009/03/03/business/03medschool.html.
249. Ibid.
250. Ornish, *Dr. Dean Ornish's Program for Reversing Heart Disease*, 53.
251. John Abramson, *Overdo$ed America: The Broken Promise of American Medicine* (New York: HarperCollins, 2004), 230–31.
252. Marcia Angell, *The Truth about the Drug Companies: How They Deceive Us and What to Do about It* (New York: Random House, 2005), 170.
253. Abramson, *Overdo$ed America*, 222.
254. Angell, *The Truth about the Drug Companies*, 169–70.
255. Ibid., 170.
256. Abramson, *Overdo$ed America*, 124.
257. Esselstyn, *Prevent and Reverse Heart Disease*, 59.
258. Michael Jacobson, "Politics 101," *Nutrition Action Healthletter*, September 2004, 2.
259. Esselstyn, *Prevent and Reverse Heart Disease*, 60.
260. Ibid.
261. Nestle, *Food Politics*, 360.
262. Ibid.
263. Ibid., 117.
264. Ibid., 119.
265. Physicians Committee for Responsible Medicine, "Farm Bill Reform," Stop Childhood Obesity Now, http://www.pcrm.org/childhoodobesity/funds.html.
266. Ibid.
267. Ibid.
268. Nestle, *Food Politics*, 361.
269. Michael Moss, "While Warning about Fat, U.S. Pushes Cheese Sales," *New York Times*, November 6, 2010, http://www.nytimes.com/2010/11/07/us/07fat.html.
270. Ibid.
271. Ibid.
272. Campbell, *The China Study*, 181–82.
273. Bill Clinton, interview by Wolf Blitzer, September 22, 2010, CNN, http://eatocracy.cnn.com/2010/09/22/clinton-plants-the-seeds-of-change-in-a-notoriously-dire-diet.

274. Tony Gonzalez, *The All-Pro Diet: Lose Fat, Build Muscle, and Live like a Champion* (New York: Rodale, 2009), 7.

275. Ibid., 4.

276. Fuhrman, *Eat to Live*, 236.

277. Robbins, *Diet for a New America*, 314–15.

278. Ibid., 315.

279. Fuhrman, *Eat to Live*, 129

280. Lyman, *Mad Cowboy*, 40.

281. Ibid, 39.

282. Robbins, *Diet for a New America*, 315.

283. Lyman, *No More Bull!*, 65.

284. Nutrition information from http://nutritiondata.self.com.

285. McDougall and McDougall, *The McDougall Plan*.

286. Dean Ornish, *Eat More, Weigh Less: Dr. Dean Ornish's Program for Losing Weight Safely while Eating Abundantly* (New York: HarperTorch, 2002), 72 (emphasis in original).

287. Campbell, *The China Study*, 244.

288. Ornish, *Eat More, Weigh Less*, 72 (emphasis in original).

289. William James, *The Principles of Psychology* (New York: Henry Holt, 1918), 1:123 (emphasis in original).

290. "Breakfast Bars, Oats, Sugar, Raisins, Coconut (Include Granola Bar)" Nutrition Data, http://nutritiondata.self.com/facts/snacks/7611/2.

291. "Egg, Whole, Cooked, Scrambled," Nutrition Data, http://nutritiondata.self.com/facts/dairy-and-egg-products/120/2. See also "Spinach, Frozen, Chopped or Leaf, Cooked, Boiled, Drained, without Salt," Nutrition Data, http://nutritiondata.self.com/facts/vegetables-and-vegetable-products/263; "Mushrooms, Cooked, Boiled, Drained, without Salt," Nutrition Data, http://nutrition-data.self.com/facts/vegetables-and-vegetable-products/2483/2.

292. Results reported in the table are based on the observations of the five MD's referenced in Chapter 1. I reviewed the concept with Dr. T. Colin Campbell after a healthy breakfast in his home, and he agreed that it was a terrific concept to help people focus on something positive and avoid the typical approach of being concerned only about what they are giving up. Dr. Campbell has often said, "The closer we get to consuming nothing but whole, plant-based foods, the better off we will be." See www.4leafprogram.com for more information.

293. McDougall, *The McDougall Program for a Healthy Heart*, 65.

294. Jeff Novick, "Principles in Practice: Label Reading," course in Cornell's Plant-Based Nutrition certificate program.

295. Michael Pollan, *In Defense of Food: An Eater's Manifesto* (New York: Penguin Press, 2008), 117.

296. "Cereals Ready-to-Eat, Kraft, Post Banana Nut Crunch Cereal," Nutrition Data, http://nutritiondata.self.com/facts/breakfast-cereals/1729/2; "Cereals Ready-to-Eat, Kraft, Post Raisin Bran Cereal," Nutrition Data, http://nutritiondata.self.com/facts/breakfast-cereals/7280/2.

297. Dr. and Mrs. Caldwell Esselstyn in lecture at the Stonington Harbor Yacht Club in Stonington, CT, on August 25, 2010.

298. Fuhrman, *Eat to Live*, 50.

299. Neal Barnard, *Eat Right, Live Longer: Using the Natural Power of Foods to Age-Proof Your Body* (New York: Three Rivers Press, 1997), 26.

300. Campbell, *The China Study*, 228.

301. Ibid., 242.

302. Schlosser, *Fast Food Nation*, 140.

303. Robbins, *The Food Revolution*, 302.

304. "Vertebrate," *New World Encyclopedia*, August 29, 2008, http://www.newworldencyclopedia.org/entry/Vertebrate.

305. Mary Brophy Marcus, "Diabetes Cases May Triple by 2050," *USA Today*, October 22, 2010, 1.

306. *Saturday Night Live*, episode aired on NBC on October 23, 2010. Meyers was referring to the latest item on the KFC menu, the "Double Down" sandwich with bacon and cheese tucked between two chicken patties.

INDEX

Tables are indicated by *t* following page number.